Yoga for Couples

Yoga for Couples

James R. Lewis
(Pundit Singh)

Illustrated by Nancy Jatko

Published by Autumn Press, Inc.,
with editorial offices at
25 Dwight Street
Brookline, Massachusetts 02146

Distributed in the United States
by Random House, Inc., and in
Canada by Random House of Canada, Ltd.

Copyright © 1979 by James R. Lewis
All rights reserved.
Library of Congress Catalog Card Number: 78-73473
ISBN: 0-394-73778-4
Printed in the United States of America
Typeset at dnh, Cambridge, Massachusetts
Illustrated by Nancy Jatko
Book design and typography by Beverly Stiskin

Table of Contents

Acknowledgments 7
Preface 8

Part I.   Tantric Yoga

Yoga and Consciousness   11
Yoga and Energy   17
Self-transcendence   23
Guidelines for Practice   28
Sadhana: Regular Practice   37

Part II.   The Exercises

Tantric Exercises   43
1. Basic Energy Awareness Techniques   45
2. Tantric Yoga Exercises   51
3. Magnetic Field Exercises   71
4. Breath Coordination Techniques   85
5. Subtle Awareness Exercises   93
6. Tantric Meditations   101
7. Group Practices   107
Glossary   110

Acknowledgments

To my first spiritual teachers—my parents

I owe a great deal to Pat Senft for her help and loving patience, and to my sister, Mae Kessemochen.

I also want to thank all the people who have helped me in preparing manuscripts about tantra over the years: Ken Meads, Debra Lightwing, Kathrine Graves, Maureen and Rick Pratt, Reen and Charles Miller, Paul Trager, Susan Triolo, Jerry Barr, and Nahum Stiskin.

Finally, I acknowledge my indebtedness to Yogi Bhajan. Although many of the techniques in this book are drawn from other traditions (notably Sufism), his teachings form the basis of my understanding of interpersonal yoga.

Preface

The term "tantric yoga" has been applied to a confusing variety of different practices and ideas. This book is a practical introduction to a specific form of tantric yoga known as "mahan tantric yoga," or "white tantric yoga." Mahan tantric is a system of interpersonal exercises and meditations which are based on the technique of gazing steadily into another person's eyes.

Interpersonal tantra has the unusual quality of being both a spiritual and a psychological technique. Viewed as a psychotherapy, tantric yoga has as its goal deepened interpersonal relationships. Viewed as a spiritual path, the goal of tantric yoga is higher consciousness.

White tantric yoga has the general purpose of transforming human relationships (relationships between personalities) into spiritual relationships (relationships between souls). At a higher level, white tantric meditations, if practiced regularly over a long period of time, will tune a person into mystical states of awareness by opening his or her higher centers of consciousness.

This book is designed to be accessible even to those with no background in yoga or meditation. (For that reason a glossary is provided at the back of the book.) Readers familiar with yoga may wish to skip over the initial two chapters on basic yoga theory.

Part I. Tantric Yoga

Yoga and Consciousness

What is Yoga?

In India the word yoga applies to a vast number of techniques and methods, all designed to raise the level of consciousness of the practitioner. The body postures that most people associate with yoga are a part of only a minority of these different systems. (Even in those yoga systems which make use of body postures, the health benefits of the exercises are considered to be of only secondary importance: serious yoga practitioners aspire to physical health only because they believe it will help them to increase their level of awareness.) Other types of yoga center on meditation—that is, mind-centering and mind-calming techniques. Body posture–type yoga can be practiced without meditation, and meditation-type yoga can be practiced without body postures, but in many yoga systems, body postures and meditation are both practiced.

The word *yoga* comes from an ancient Sanskrit word meaning "union." All of the different methods that are referred to as "yoga" share the common goal of uniting the individual with a higher reality. This higher reality is called by different names, depending on the particular consciousness-raising system: the True Self, God, the Oversoul, the Higher Self, et cetera. The "union" takes place in a state of higher consciousness, a state of increased awareness. Again, there are many different names for this state: *samadhi, nirvana,* Christ consciousness, *satori*, cosmic consciousness, enlightenment, et cetera. In actuality, of course, the individual is always linked with this higher reality: the process of reaching a higher level of consciousness is the process of becoming aware of this link.

One of the best ways for discussing higher consciousness is in terms of levels of awareness. Normally we experience only a limited aspect of reality. But there is a range of consciousness available to us that is so much more aware (or more "awake") than our normal state of consciousness that if we could tune into these higher levels, they would make our everyday waking state appear like sleep. When a person "wakes up" to higher consciousness, it is so much more real than the everyday state that it makes normal "waking" consciousness appear like a dream. The realization is so radical that, from the perspective of higher consciousness, our everyday concerns seem trivial.

This is not to say, however, that our everyday experience of the world is a total illusion. Rather, it is only a very limited perspective on reality. When we tune into higher levels of consciousness, we experience it as a change of perspective enabling us to "see" more of reality.

Yoga Psychology

Another way to understand the idea of higher consciousness is in terms of yoga psychology. Classical yoga psychology and traditional western psychology bear very little resemblance to each other. Traditional western psychotherapy deals with the question, Given an *abnormal* individual, how can s/he be helped to become *normal*? Yoga takes the approach, Given a *normal* individual, how can s/he evolve into a *supernormal* person?

The starting point of yoga psychology is the idea that we can distinguish between our true, real self (the "soul") and our normal, everyday self (the "personality"). This yoga distinction is very similar to the psyche-persona distinction of the ancient Greeks: The outer, publicly visible self (the *persona* or personality) is the mask of the real, inner self (the *psyche* or soul).

In the context of yoga, the word for "soul," *atman*, refers to the essence of the person—to that part which never changes; each individual's center of pure consciousness. "Personality," *ahamkara*, on the other hand, refers to that collection of habitual patterns of thought, feelings, and mannerisms which most people normally think of as their "self" (*ahamkara* traditionally refers only to the "sense of self" which is the foundation of the personality). According to yoga psychology, our central problem is that we identify ourselves with our personality and either forget or else don't know that each of us is something more than just a personality.

This problem—along with a proposed solution—was well expressed in the *Yoga Sutras* of Patanjali (composed about 200 B.C.):

> Yoga is the restraint or stilling of the modifications of the mind. [These "modifications" are thoughts, feelings, perceptions, et cetera.]
> When the mind can be thus restrained, a person can become one with his own true self.
> Otherwise, he will mistakenly identify himself with his thoughts, feelings, and perceptions.

What this means, in simple language, is that normally we are so involved with whatever we are doing and thinking that we have forgotten who we really are. Further, what we need to do, in order to get back in touch with ourselves, is to stop whatever we are doing and just "be" for a while. This is, of course, an oversimplification, but it does convey the general idea of what is being expressed by these three aphorisms.

Beyond the Personality

According to yoga psychology, we can distinguish consciousness from the objects of consciousness. The objects of consciousness are anything of which we can be aware (thoughts, feelings, perceptions, etc.). Pure consciousness (or pure awareness) is that intangible "something" which distinguishes the state of consciousness from that of unconsciousness. According to the analysis offered by yoga psychology, pure consciousness is identical with our True Self, or center.

The objects in the mind might be thought of as images on a movie screen, with our own everyday life story as the plot. The awareness (pure consciousness), on the other hand, is like the individual who is watching the movie. As long as we remain immersed in our own personal drama, we will continue to identify ourselves with our life drama and will never be able to realize that we are something more than our everyday "actor" self.

Another, more traditional, image is that of a lake (the mind substance), which normally has many disturbed waves (the objects in the mind), caused by currents and winds (emotions, impressions, etc.). When the lake of the mind becomes calm through meditation, the silt settles out and we can finally see the bottom—that is, our true self.

Soul and Self

Soul and personality are not discrete entities, but two poles of the one self. A more accurate way of visualizing the soul-personality relationship is as the center and the circumference of a circle (figure 1).

For purposes of meditation or therapy, a similar and even better image is that of a hurricane or a tornado. As long as we remain immersed in everyday life (the realm of personality), we are going to be continually blown about by the stormy events in our life drama, and by our reactions to these events. If we can become "centered" (via such techniques as meditation and yoga), then we will find ourselves in the calm, clear eye of the storm (the level of the soul) and need no longer be swept along by external events.

The expressions "spiritual growth" and "spiritual path" refer to the long journey upon which the individual must embark before s/he can become attuned to the soul. Thus, a "spiritual technique" is any technique which helps us to make this inward journey. And to be "spiritual" in everyday life means to relate to life in a centered way.

Figure 1.

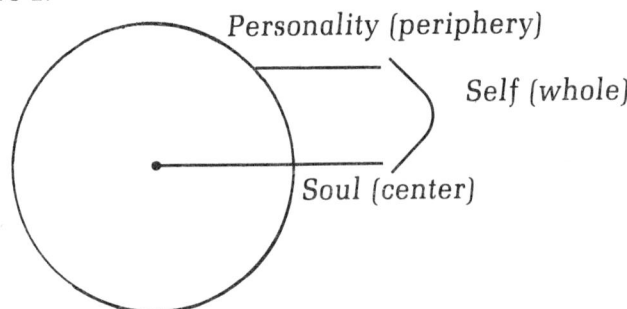

Psychology and Personality

Traditional psychotherapies (such as Freudian psychology) deal with those problems that prevent the individual from functioning in society. But this type of theoretical model, which was borrowed from medical science, is severely limited, and of little use to those who are dissatisfied and feel the urge to search for a deeper meaning in life. Thus, especially since the middle of this century, new, humanistic psychologies have been evolved which try to include the deeper aspects of the human person.

"Humanistic psychology" tries to understand the personality in such a way as to emphasize its growing, evolving, and creative characteristics. It goes one step beyond traditional medical psychology by pointing out that there are stages of psychological growth possible *beyond* an adjustment to society. But humanistic psychology still focuses on the personality and only very rarely takes the further step of including the concept of a center or soul which is beyond the personality.

Western psychology emphasizes the personality and eastern psychology emphasizes the soul. However, since the soul and the personality are not two separate entities, the two approaches necessarily overlap rather than simply complement each other.

Spiritual Techniques as Therapy

Soul psychology can contribute to personality psychology. In general, the various spiritual techniques (meditation and yoga) allow the individual to take a step back from her/his personality, so that, from this more detached perspective, s/he can gain a more objective self-understanding. The individual can then work more clearly with negative personality patterns which limit growth.

Most of our greatest problems originate as part of a psychological defense mechanism. As a result, whenever we try to modify or work out one of these problems, we reactivate the anxiety that gave birth to the defense mechanism in the first place. This process hinders change, and consequently it usually takes a long time to work out a negative pattern. Almost everyone has had the experience of understanding—abstractly—how he or she is hung-up and yet being unable to overcome an old habit pattern.

The practice of yoga—and particularly yoga meditation—tunes us into the calm, clear, peaceful center of our being. In the early stages of practice, this peace is usually felt only during the yoga session itself, but after an extended period of regular practice, this tranquility begins to pervade all of our activities. As this peace becomes more and more established, we are able to bring our problems to the surface with less anxiety, and thus modify old patterns with greater ease. Instead of dealing with the problem as part of an emotionally charged defense mechanism, we can deal with it as a mechanical, bad habit. Greater objectivity and lessened anxiety are the primary psychotherapeutic benefits that can be derived from spiritual techniques.

Yoga and Energy

The concept of a personal energy field or energy "body" is basic to yogic theory. In the tantric exercises two people blend their energy fields and try to become aware of specific interpersonal energy flows.

The Subtle Body

Classical yoga theory holds that an energy field or body surrounds and interpenetrates the physical body. Western mystical terminology refers to this subtle body as the "etheric body" and to the subtle energy as "etheric energy." Current research into phenomena such as Kirlian photography and acupuncture tends to corroborate the existence of the subtle body.

Yoga theory is in fact very similar to acupuncture theory. The Indians and the Chinese both attribute to the energy body a definite "anatomy," with energy channels (*nadis* or meridians) which conduct subtle forces (*prana* or *chi*) to the various parts of the body.

Yoga is the science of clearing and strengthening each part of the subtle body until it is able to handle more potent energy flows. The increased energy can then be used to reach higher levels of awareness (figure 2).

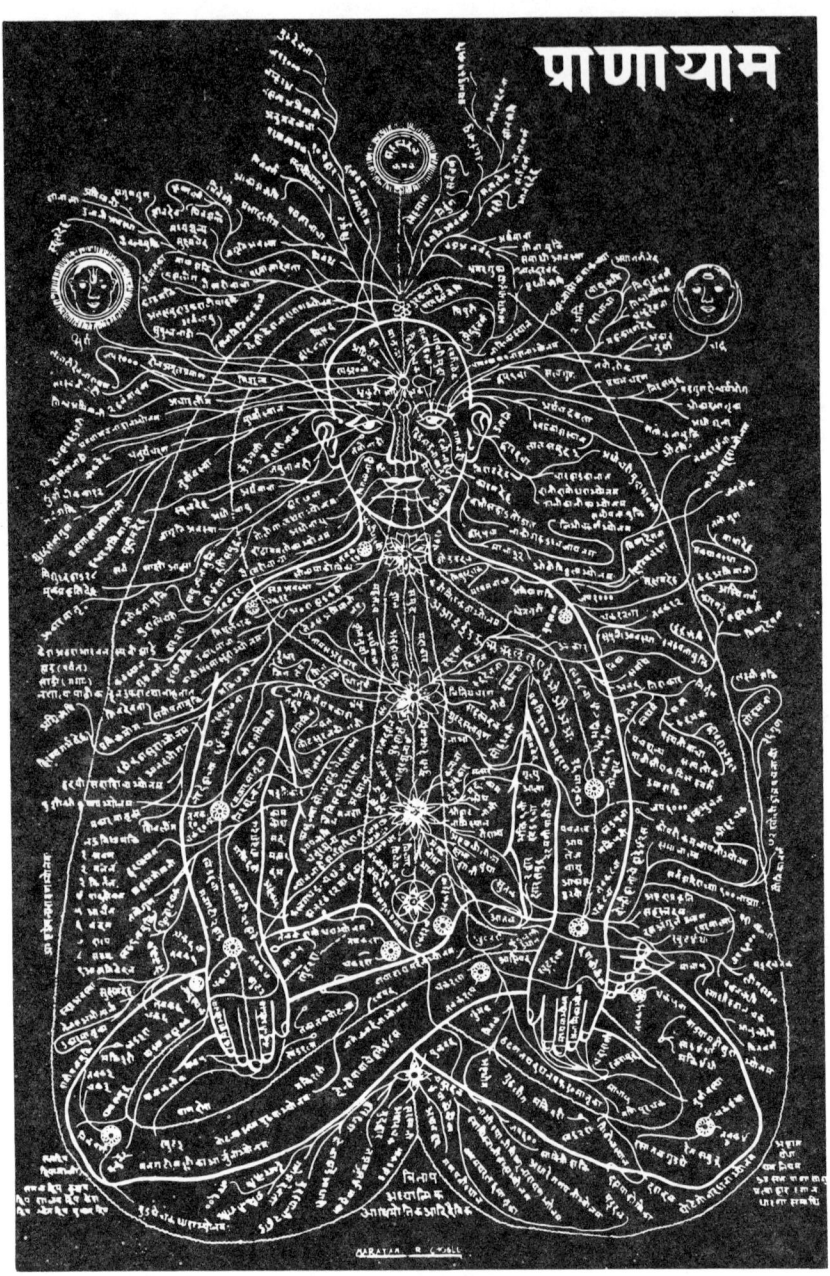

Figure 2. Traditional diagram of the anatomy of the subtle body. The words labeling the various nadis and chakras are in Sanskrit script; the title in the upper right hand corner says "energy control" (pranayam).

18   Yoga for Couples

The Chakras

The subtle anatomy has energy centers which regulate the flow of *prana* in the body. The major centers lie along a channel which goes from the base of the spine to the crown of the head. These *chakras* ("wheels")[1] are simultaneously centers of energy and centers of consciousness.

As centers of energy, chakras could be compared with electrical transformers: they transmute the one basic energy that runs through the body into different forms, so that it may perform a variety of different functions.

There are seven major chakras. The first chakra (at the base of the spine) is the source of stronger than normal energy currents. When this energy generator is completely "switched on," current flows up a central energy channel (which corresponds with the spine) and activates the higher centers. When strong energy is directed into the head chakras, we experience higher levels of consciousness. Many years of practice must be accomplished before the energy can be activated completely, because the entire subtle body system must be purified and strengthened in order to be able to handle the stronger energy flows. The higher chakras are rarely active in the average person. We might understand them as being analogues to electrical appliances to which current is not flowing—that is, ordinarily they are not "turned on."

Although the chakras are not physical, the subtle body does interpenetrate the physical body; thus, the chakras can be located by referring to areas of the physical body (figure 3).

Male-Female Polarities

Each person is a mixture of both positive and negative energy—yang and yin chi. Each individual is a blend of both male and female (positive and negative) energies, but males tend to be more yang (positive) and females tend to be more yin (negative). Since energy fields between people of opposite sexes blend more easily, tantric yoga usually involves a male-female couple; however, the techniques are also effective with couples of the same sex.

[1] Chakras appear to those endowed with psychic sight as spheres or wheels of light.

Figure 3. The Seven Major Chakras

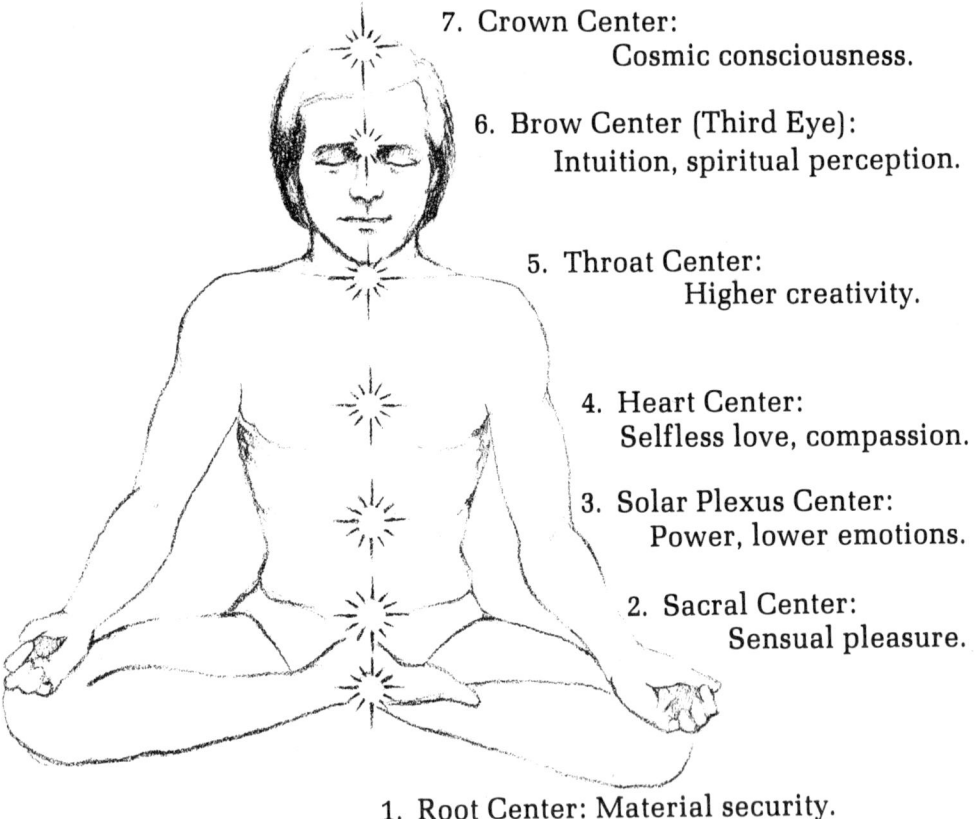

7. Crown Center:
    Cosmic consciousness.

6. Brow Center (Third Eye):
    Intuition, spiritual perception.

5. Throat Center:
    Higher creativity.

4. Heart Center:
    Selfless love, compassion.

3. Solar Plexus Center:
    Power, lower emotions.

2. Sacral Center:
    Sensual pleasure.

1. Root Center: Material security.

Interpersonal Energy Flows

Energy flows in and out of the body more easily at certain points and areas. In interpersonal yoga, only certain of the larger and more useful high-conductivity areas are used. Energy flows easily through the chakras, of course, but this is a far more subtle experience; in order to be aware of it, one usually needs some prior practice of yoga/meditation disciplines. The more basic tantric techniques utilize contact between the bottoms of the feet, the palms of the hands, and the fingertips, all of which are especially good conductors.

Energy also flows between the eyes. In most tantric exercises the partners gaze steadily into each other's eyes. During eye contact, an energy exchange occurs.

Blending Energy Fields

Much of the purpose of yoga exercise is to strengthen and clear out the subtle energy body so that it can handle more powerful energy flows, thereby activating the higher centers and tuning into higher states of consciousness. The chief advantage of white tantric yoga is that more energy is available for raising the level of consciousness. When a flow is established between two people, the energy that circulates between them is the combined energy of both individuals, rather than the individual energies of either. (This can be compared with the blending of two atoms into one molecule: two separate particles become one larger particle with a stronger combined energy.)

This reinforcement of energy enhances all of the purposes of yoga. By running the combined energy currents from two people through different parts of the energy body (during different tantric positions), the subtle energy channels (nadis) are being purified in a much more powerful way than they would be for the individual practicing yoga. Thus, the process of breaking down energy blockages and strengthening the circuitry of the subtle body is considerably accelerated.

In the yogic schema, current flows from positive to negative. According to yoga theory, the right side of the body is predominantly positive, whereas the left side is predominantly negatively charged. In simple energy awareness techniques using the hands and the feet, the right side of one person's body (right hand or right foot) is brought near—or into contact with—the partner's left side. This positioning occurs naturally when two individuals face each other. With groups in a circle, energy flows into each person's left side and out through the right side, so that the energy moves throughout the entire circle in a circular pattern. In both situations a closed circuit of subtle energy is created.

Self-transcendence

Very often seekers on the spiritual path get caught up in narcissistic self-preoccupation: "I want to get it together," "I want to be enlightened," "I want to reach *samadhi*"—the focus always being "I." During many stages of spiritual growth such preoccupation is perhaps necessary, but it can become a trap. Part of the purpose of white tantric yoga is to help us break out of our egocentrism by expanding our spiritual practices beyond the narrow boundaries of the self.

Oneness

At the initial stages of white tantric practice, practitioners are still tuned in to a personality level. But as the practice deepens, they begin to go beyond the facial features, beyond eye color, and thoughts of what the other person is thinking. The eyes truly become the windows of the soul. This is a profound experience, difficult to describe without poetry.

As they relax into an interpersonal meditation, the energy fields become more and more blended, until the two individuals become literally two bodies sitting in one field of energy. There is no definite place where one subtle body ends and the other one begins. This blending requires that the partners sit steadily for quite some time, and that they be able to lower their psychological defenses, which tend to produce energy "walls" that block the flow of energy.

When the blending has become deep enough, the partners are able to touch each other at a soul level. Again, this is difficult to describe in words; yet it is a definite experience. White tantric yoga is one of the few spiritual practices that has as its goal the joining of two individuals at their deepest spiritual levels. The mystical idea of Oneness ceases to be an abstract concept; instead, it becomes a direct experience.

As each person meditates into the other's eyes, the eyes become *yantras* (meditation diagrams or mandalas), drawing each person deeper and deeper into the other person; simultaneously each is drawn deep within him- or herself. Ultimately, both have the experience of being one soul in two bodies. Metaphorically, their situation is comparable to a house at night in which there is one light burning: from the outside the light is seen shining out of many windows, and thus it appears to be many different lights, but if we change our perspective and go into the house, we discover that there is really only one light source. Similarly, there is only one consciousness, and we are its many windows.

The regular practice of tantric techniques can help us to begin to glimpse each individual's spiritual self. In the midst of an ordinary conversation, suddenly our eyes will meet, and we will briefly "touch" at a far deeper level of communion than is usual.

Beyond the Self

The white tantric exercises themselves require self-transcendence. In order for each individual to rise in consciousness during a practice, s/he is compelled to relate to the partner's state of consciousness. The more one transcends the self and focuses instead on helping the partner to experience an elevated state of awareness, the higher both people will become. There is a see-saw effect, and gradually the level of consciousness of both partners is raised.

The exercises also require physical "self-transcendence." The longer, deeper, more meditative exercises, in particular, require one to sit perfectly still for long periods of time; any movement will disturb the experience for the partner. Continually sacrificing one's own comfort for the other person's sake helps one to transcend the narrowness of self-preoccupation.

Psychological Dimensions

The chakras are at once energy centers and centers of consciousness; each center represents a particular mental state.

The three lower centers represent the worldly energies associated with survival, desire, and power. The three upper centers correspond to states of consciousness in which the individual relates to planes of reality that transcend this world. The middle center, at the heart, is a key chakra because it balances the upper and the lower centers. The heart represents compassion, love, and selfless service—the spirit (upper three centers) in relationship to the world (lower three centers). The image of "opening the heart" refers very concretely to the experience of feeling energy flowing up and opening the heart center.

Tantric yoga ultimately aims to lift the awareness to the sixth and seventh chakras, but to do so the tantric techniques must first work on the heart center to break up the *samskaras* (blockages) that keep the energy from flowing up, through, and past the heart. White tantric yoga, and specifically heart center techniques, are very powerful tools for breaking up heart chakra blockages.

The idea of tantric yoga is to tune in to a very deep place, yet not an intense place. (This distinction may seem subtle, but it is important: often people become overly concerned with the mystique of tantric yoga and expect some strange, mystical experience.) During practice, it is quite all right to smile or even to laugh. Smiling and laughing both open the heart, which is a necessity in this form of tantra.

Many people are uncomfortable about physical contact and prolonged eye contact. Going through the white tantric experience can help them to work through this discomfort—by helping them to put personalities aside and relate, without anxieties or expectations, at a deep spiritual level.

Tantric Therapy

The spiritual quest and the psychological quest both attempt to overcome negative personality patterns associated with interpersonal relationships. By increasing self-objectivity and lessening anxiety, yoga and meditation (in general) and tantric yoga practice (in particular) help us to work out problems in our interpersonal relationships. From the viewpoint of humanistic psychology, better human relationships are those which are more authentic, involving less manipulation or game playing. When practiced properly, white tantric yoga takes one beyond the game playing level, even if only temporarily. Of course, an individual or a couple can still play games with subtle facial expressions, but as long as the major facilitator of game playing, the mouth, is shut, they can at least obtain a glimpse of what it is like to relate without games.

In order for white tantric yoga to begin to break up game-playing tendencies, it must be practiced regularly, for a reasonably long period of time. Only when one has become established in the security of the soul level can one drop psychological defense mechanisms. Then it becomes possible to effect changes in the personality from the inside out.

Spiritual Marriage

The special usefulness of white tantric yoga lies in the area of improving male-female relationships, such as marriage, by transforming them into truly spiritual relationships. Tantric techniques added to a couple's daily *sadhana* (spiritual practices) will permit them to share the deepest aspect of conscious growth. Couples who want to work out a specific set of problems will find that tantric techniques help them to be more objective and less emotional about the patterns of relating that are generating the problems. Couples who want to improve and deepen their relationship will find that practicing tantric yoga regularly will gradually enable them to relate to each other in a progressively more authentic way. Couples who want to grow together spiritually will find that tantric yoga allows them to tune into each other at a soul level.

Human beings operate on many different levels, and a joining can occur on one level or on several levels simultaneously. On the physical level, a mutual attraction expresses itself as sexual desire, but in physical union one's desire for a feeling of oneness can only be satisfied temporarily. Even mutual love and understanding—union at an emotional/mental (personality) level—can be frustrating because it is incomplete, and still subject to fluctuations of mood and circumstances; it fails to penetrate to the deepest level of pure spirit. The experience that white tantric yoga ultimately aims at is union at the soul level, completely transcending personalities. Only at a spiritual level can the experience of union ever be completely satisfying.

Again, tantra allows us to become consciously aware of a link that has been there all along. We are all part of the whole universe, but perhaps unconsciously so. The highest potentiality of marriage is that it can be a vehicle for achieving conscious union, or yoga.

Guidelines for Practice

Breathing

Breathing techniques are of vital importance in yoga: by changing the way be breathe, we can change the way that energy flows in the body. In normal, natural breathing ("diaphragm" breathing), the abdomen extends during inhalation and sinks back toward the spine upon exhalation. In the contemporary view, however, a protruding stomach is considered "ugly," so most of us keep our stomachs constantly pulled in; we breathe with the upper chest. The constant tension thus created disturbs mental calm. It also lowers the vitality (thus paving the way for disease), by restricting the energy flow of the body.

Yogic breathing is called *pranayama*. The term denotes control or restraint *(yama)* of the subtle energy *(prana)*. Yogic exercises make use of both long, deep breathing and short, rapid breathing. It helps, initially, to become adept at diaphragm breathing.

To experiment with the different breathing techniques, lie on the back. Place one hand on the very upper part of the chest and the other on the stomach, over the navel. Practice normal breathing (always breathing through the nose) by causing the belly to rise on the inhale and sink back down on the exhale. The upper chest should rise only slightly, if it moves at all.

To practice long, deep breathing, inhale and cause the stomach to rise, and then continue the inhalation so that the chest also rises. (They rise in a wave motion: stomach first, then chest.) On the exhalation let both sink down together, or else let the stomach sink down first. Practice this type of exaggerated breathing every day for a week or two until it can be done automatically.

Powerful, rapid breathing is the best type of breathing for clearing subtle nerve channels and for charging up the energy field. Inhale and cause the belly to rise. Jerk the muscles quickly back towards the back to force the air out, then inhale naturally. The breath is short, not deep. Once the breath pattern is established, build up the speed to one breath per second. This type of breathing is called *kapalabhati*.

Over time (several weeks to several months) build up the breath to three breaths per second, forcing both the inhalation and the exhalation with the diaphragm. This method of breathing is called *bhastrika*.

Breath coordination is important for some of the techniques. Couples should inhale and exhale together, or else breathe in "reversed" coordination: one person inhales as the other exhales. Both methods allow the energy fields to blend together more easily and more completely, by putting the polarity changes on a similar "schedule." The reversed coordination is especially useful for techniques in which energy is sent back and forth between the partners.

Posture

A straight back is essential during yoga meditation. ("Straight" means holding the body erect; it does not mean eliminating the natural curvature of the spine.) When the back is bent, it hinders the flow of the energy to the higher centers.

A cross-legged pose is the preferred position for meditation, because it neutralizes to a certain extent the energy flows in the lower part of the body, thus allowing the pranic energy to become concentrated in the higher centers of consciousness. An alternative is the *vajrasan* position, in which the heels are bent slightly outwards so that one is sitting partially on the side of the feet.

One should sit on as soft a surface as possible. (There are absolutely no spiritual benefits to be derived from sitting on a hard surface: the more comfortable one is, the easier it is to concentrate.) Sitting on a cushion or on a pillow, with the crossed legs resting on a surface lower than the rump, helps one to maintain a straight back without straining. It is also good to do yoga and meditation on an insulating material such as a wool blanket.

Movement

There are some adjustments that one must make at first in order to "settle in," but after that, one must go beyond the little discomforts and forcefully resist moving. Circulation in the legs will slow down after ten minutes or so, but resist movement even then (this partial restriction of the circulation can be maintained for over an hour without any negative results). The discomfort will be less if the body is kept still rather than fidgeting. Also resist itching. Even if most of the exercise is spent resisting the urge to move, this should be done.

Should the legs or back become sore, it may help to relax between exercises. Partners may wish to lie down, with either heads or feet touching.

Hand Locks

Because of the large energy current which constantly flows in and out of the body through the hands, any change in the position of the hands or the fingers will alter the way in which prana flows throughout the entire energy body. The importance of the hand position gave rise to a system of *mudras*, or "hand locks."

The Venus lock (figure 4) is a double fist in which the right thumb tip is pressed into the fleshy part of the palm at the base of the left thumb (the mount of Venus). The left thumb is pressed into the fleshy part of the right hand where the base of the thumb and the forefinger join. Fingers interlock so that the right index finger is on top of the left index finger. This lock establishes a very deep balance between the positive and negative pranas (*prana* and *apana*) of the body.

In the finger lock (figure 5) the fingers of each hand are curled, as if holding a pipe, and the hands are hooked together. The hands should be open enough so that the palms show. One hand should face in toward the body, the other outward.

When one applies tension to a finger lock (by trying to pull the hands apart), prana will begin to concentrate around the hands. If the palms are open (as they should be), the energy will then flow out into that part of the aura surrounding the hands and "charge" it.

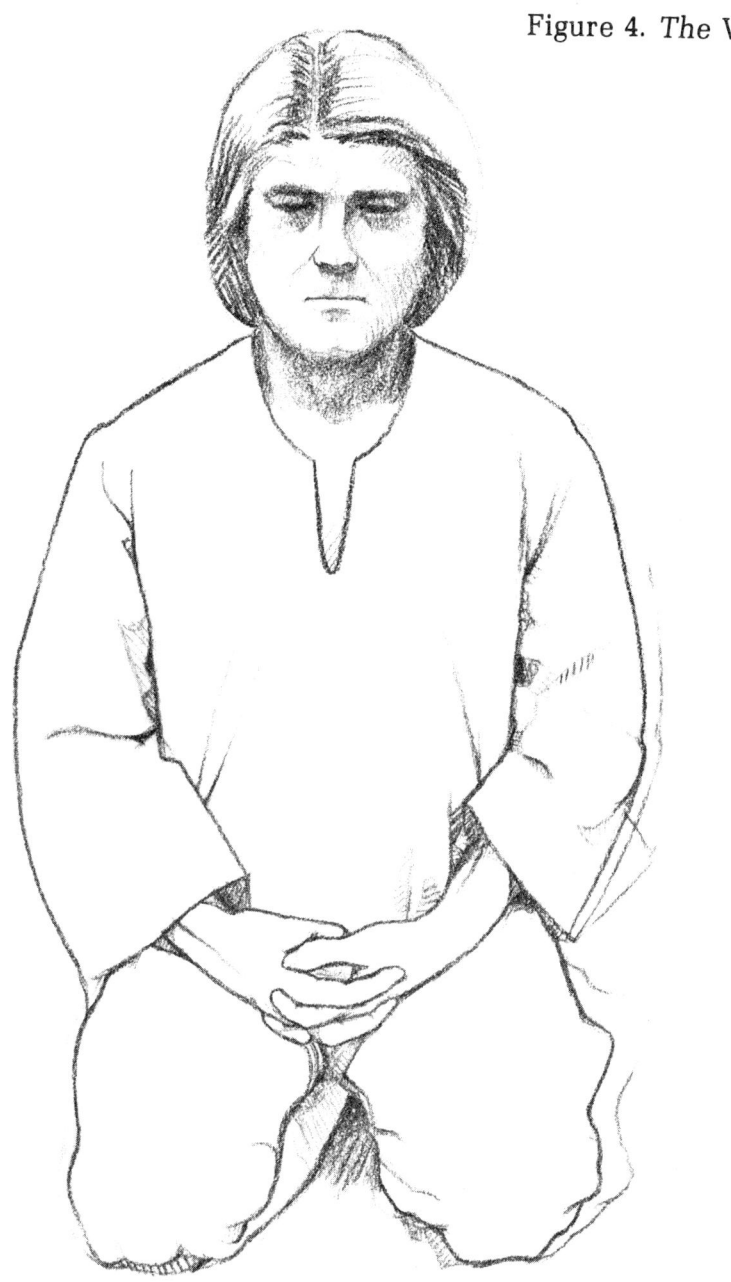

Figure 4. *The Venus Lock*

Figure 5. The Finger Lock

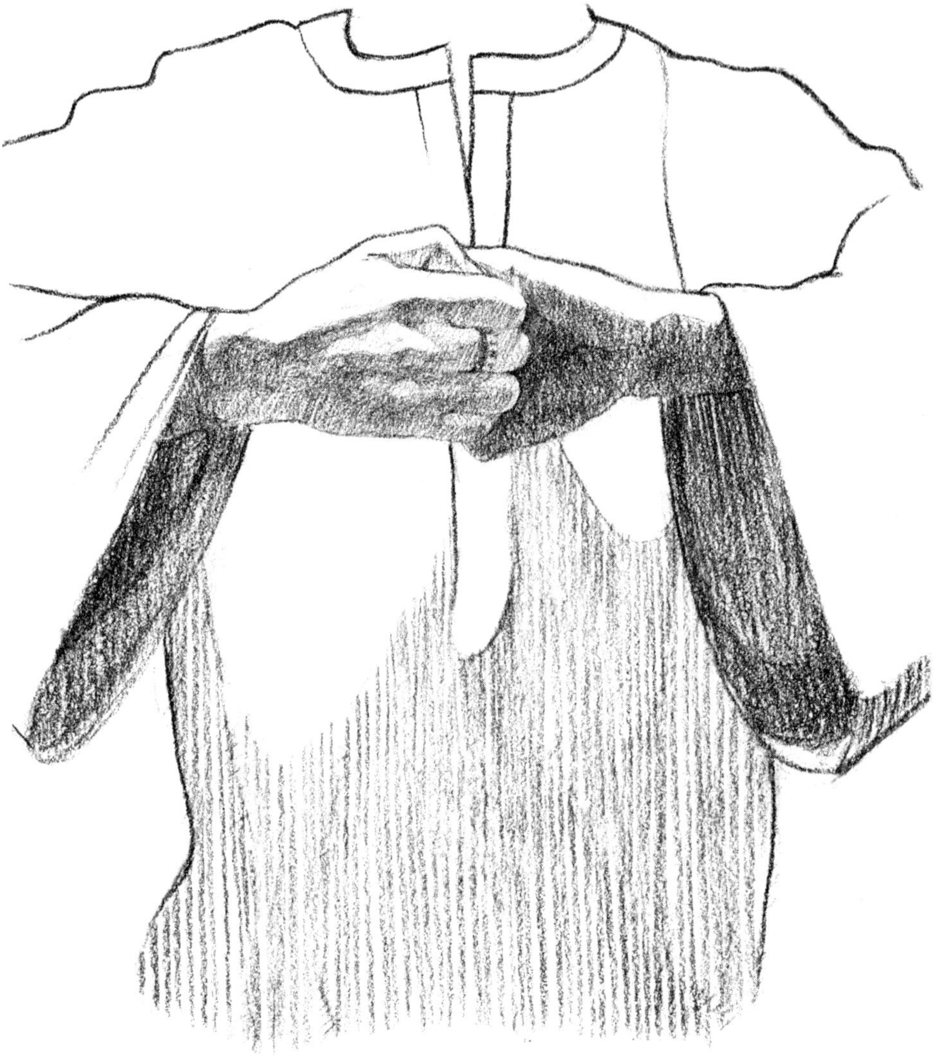

Mental Direction of Energy

Energy follows the direction of the attention. A mind powerful enough can cause even physical objects to move; however, usually only very strong and developed individuals can mentally control matter. Subtle energy, on the other hand, is much closer to mind substance (manas) than are physical objects; thus, even those with relatively weak concentration can direct energy to a degree.

The method for making use of this principle is to reproduce in the imagination the subjective sensations of subtle energy currents. At the most basic level subtle energy has a "tingling" feeling or sometimes a tangible "magnetic" feeling.

The feeling of magnetic polarity occurs when the palms are brought close together (without touching) and moved back and forth slightly. This produces a sensation which is similar to the sensation felt when two magnets are held, one in each hand, and moved back and forth near each other.

During exercises where the palms, fingertips, or soles of the feet are brought into contact, imagining a feeling of tingling sensations on the area of contact will help to cause energy to flow across that area. Also, imagining a right-to-left flow (from one partner's right side to the other partner's left side) will further stimulate the current. After a short period of contact, the couple will almost always begin to feel the tingling sensation. Imagining a warm heat sensation also helps to stimulate the flow.

To increase the effectiveness of many practices, try imagining the energy flowing through the body—either by feeling it flow as a fluid current or else by visualizing it as liquid light flowing through the body.

Eye Contact

Once the gaze is locked in, don't break it for the duration of the exercise: this is vital, because breaking the gaze can disrupt the partner's concentration and prevent the energy flow from becoming strong enough to allow the couple to tune into a deep level.

Ideally, each partner looks straight into the other person's face: one's right eye looks into the partner's left eye, and one's left eye looks into the partner's right eye. To do so, one must let the partner's face split into two images. When this occurs, allow the right eye of one image to blend into the left eye of the other image. You will then see three eyes and be looking into the center eye.

If this is not possible, one should look into the right eye of a male, the left eye of a female. Do not shift the gaze back and forth from one eye to the other.

One should also try to blink as little as possible. Sometimes it is necessary to blink, but it disturbs the energy which is flowing between the eyes. Don't worry if the eyes water—this is actually very cleansing.

During prolonged gazing the partner's face will seem to change totally. Most of these "changes" are the result of visual afterimages, but sometimes we actually see part of the other person's energy field, or perhaps get a glimpse of the partner's past lifetimes. These effects are helpful at first, in that they stimulate enough interest so that we tend to keep our attention absorbed in gazing. But after a certain length of time, one must focus in on the deeper experience of the eyes, rather than on the peripheral face changes.

Some people find prolonged eye contact difficult—perhaps because they are afraid that it will reveal hidden thoughts and feelings. This fear is unfounded. In tantric yoga contact occurs on a spiritual rather than psychological level. Occasionally we may be able to tell what is going on inside the partner's head, but not very clearly and not very often. That the contact is "safe" should be borne in mind; otherwise, our insecurities may prevent us from lowering our defensive energy patterns.

Conscious Blending

When one first practices tantric yoga, the ego will obviously tend to resist the experience of egolessness, by remaining stuck at the psychological/personality level. As the partners' energy fields blend, one needs to surrender more and more. At the beginning of a tantric technique one should relax and remember that it is not a contest of wills. It helps to remember that one is surrendering to the partner's spirit rather than to his or her personality.

Try to go beyond facial features and thoughts about the partner's physical appearance. Leave behind associations with the partner's personality and thoughts about what the other person is thinking. Any of these kinds of thoughts or associations keep the techniques from going deeper.

Relate to the gazing as a meditation in which the eyes are mandalas. In the same way that a mandala continually pulls the observer's awareness deeper and deeper into its geometrical patterns, the partner's eyes can become whirlpools that pull one in. Simultaneously, one should go deep within oneself. The idea is for the couple to experience being one soul in two bodies.

Tantric Exercises

Table 1.

A. Basic Energy Awareness Techniques
    1. *Magnetic Energy Awareness*
    2. *Energy Flow through Fingertips*
        2V (variation). *Energy Flow through Palms*
    3. *Energy Flow through Saturn Fingers*
    4. *Energy Flow through Soles, Sitting Up*
        4V. *Energy Flow through Soles, Lying Down*
    5. *Hold Shoulders*

B. Tantric Yoga Exercises
    6. *Spinal Flex, Legs Crossed*
        6V. *Spinal Flex on Heels*
    7. *Squats*
    8. *Crow Pose*
    9. *Rising Vajrasan*
    10. *Seesaw*
    11. *Moving Cobra Pose*
        11V. *Stationary Cobra Pose*

C. Magnetic Field Exercises
    12. *Tricuti Kriya, Rapid*
        12V. *Tricuti Kriya, Slow*
    13. *Hands Palmed, Arms Straight*

14. Hands Clasped, Lean Back
15. Arms Up 60°
    15V. Arms Up 90°
16. Back to Back, Arms Up 60°
17. Legs Up inside Arms
    17V. Legs Up outside Arms
18. Fingerlock at Heart
    18V. Finger Lock over Crown

D. Breath Coordination Techniques
   19. Arica Breath Coordination
   20. Finger-to-Knee Breath Coordination
   21. Stand Back to Back
       21V. Sit Back to Back

E. Subtle Awareness Techniques
   22. Hand to Heart
       22V. Finger to Third Eye
   23. Crown Centers Touching
       23V. Crown Centers Apart
   24. Third Eyes Touching
   25. Heart Beam
       25 1st V. Heart Beam, Gaze at Chest
       25 2nd V. Heart Beam, Visualization
       25 3rd V. Heart Beam, with Coordinated Breathing
   26. Third Eye Beam
       26 1st V. Third Eye Beam, Visualization
       26 2nd V. Third Eye Beam, Gaze at Forehead
       26 3rd V. Third Eye Beam, with Coordinated Breathing

F. Tantric Meditations
   27. Meditate Face to Face
       27V. Meditate Holding Hands
   28. Meditate Back to Back
       28V. Spinal Heat
   29. Meditate with Mantra

G. Group Practices
   30. Stand in a Circle
   31. Heads Together in a Circle
   32. Sit in a Circle
       32 1st V. Meditate in a Circle
       32 2nd V. Gaze across a Circle

Sadhana: Regular Practice

The repetition of any activity will produce a habit, whether that habit is good or bad. Old habits can be broken, in time, by imposing a new habit on top of an old habit. For a length of time there is a "tension" between the old and new pattern, and then, if we persevere, the old rhythm is entirely replaced by the new one. This, in a very oversimplified form, is the understanding that underlies *sadhana*, or regular practice.

In a tantric yoga sadhana, the old habits that we want to break up are our problems with interpersonal relationships: anxieties, negative feelings, game-playing, egocentrism, et cetera. The new pattern that we wish to superimpose is the habit of looking at everyone else in an understanding, empathetic way, as a fellow soul. This goal, the goal of transforming the inauthentic personality into a spiritual personality, encompasses the first two stages of tantric sadhana.

The other goal of tantric yoga is for us to become established in that state of consciousness where we *know* (rather than just believe) that everybody is part of the One Soul. In this state we experience cosmic consciousness. When this goal is attained, then we have reached the third state of sadhana.

The traditional outline of the three stages of sadhana is as follows:

1. *Sadhana* (stage of discipline or effort)
2. *Radhana* (stage of attitude or habit)
3. *Prabhupati* (stage of mastery)

During the first stage, we are striving (and many times struggling) to establish a new pattern in our lives. During the second stage, we have been so successful that our new pattern no longer requires effort; it is a part of us. During this stage we may also begin to have "cosmic" experiences, but they are usually fleeting and not under our control. It is only in the third that we *are* cosmic; we can consciously enter the soul level, consciously return to the personality level, and live our everyday life from our center.

Practice for Beginners

Those who are just starting tantric yoga should concern themselves more with becoming comfortable with the technique than with trying to do the exercises in a technically perfect way.

Begin by working with the basic technique of tantric yoga, eye contact (#27), for 5–10 minutes. Afterwards pause for a while, give each other some feedback, and then resume eye contact.

Once you have worked with the eye contact long enough to get over initial anxieties and expectations, move on to section A, "Basic Energy Awareness Techniques." This set of exercises is designed (1) to serve as a basis for subtler techniques (such as those in section E) and (2) to allow the couple to blend their auras consciously.

In exercise 1, "Magnetic Energy Awareness," experience the energy first as individuals, for 1–2 minutes, and then try to establish the feeling of magnetic polarity between the partners, by focusing the attention primarily on the hands. After several minutes most people will feel something, but do not worry if nothing happens the first time: continue to experiment with the rest of the techniques in section A until "energy" becomes a perceptible reality rather than an abstract concept. This will usually take only a few practice sessions.

Intermediate Practice

The most rewarding exercises for relative beginners, in addition to those in section A, are exercises #19, 22, 24, and 27V. For the irregular practitioner to gain the most basic benefits of tantric yoga practice, these exercises, plus a few others, should be sufficient. (This initial set is also a good body of techniques to draw on if one wishes to introduce someone to tantric yoga.) A series of a half-dozen can be constructed from this basic set, according to the preference of the couple. It is advisable to progress from basic to more subtle exercises, and to intersperse techniques in which the legs are extended among techniques in which the legs are crossed (to allow the circulation to return to the legs).

Systematic Practice

Systematic work with tantric yoga presupposes a familiarity with the basics and a desire for regular practice.

The techniques in section A are purely introductory: they can be dispensed with after a certain point. How long it takes to leave the introductory stage and to begin the systematic practice stage should be left to the judgment of each couple, but the couple should not rush the transition.

Sections B through F constitute a progression, and the order of these sections constitutes the basic framework for a regular set. Sections B and C are preparatory: B is designed to "tune up" the physical body (by increasing circulation in the legs and flexibility in the spine), C to charge and balance the aura. Section D blends the couple's energy fields. Sections E and F introduce deep meditations which allow the couple to tune in to the soul level: the techniques in section E establish a very subtle awareness of energy and open the higher centers, breaking up blockages; the meditations in section F are designed to enhance cosmic consciousness and the experience of one soul in two bodies.

A minimal systematic set should be constructed according to the following abstract guideline:

    From section B[1]: one exercise for the spine, one exercise for the legs
    From section C: at least one exercise for charging the aura
    From section D: one breath coordination technique

[1] Regular hatha yoga may be substituted for these exercises.

From section E: one heart center technique, one third eye technique, and, optionally, one crown center technique
From section F: one meditation

A minimum set consists of seven exercises. The first six exercises can be done for a minimum of 3 minutes each, and the last meditation for a minimum of 10 minutes, making a total of a little less than half an hour. Daily practice is preferred, but sessions three or four times a week are sufficient to be considered regular practice.

Example of a minimal set

Table 2a.

	Time	Area Affected
1. Spinal Flex, Legs Crossed (#6)	3 minutes	spine
2. Rising Vajrasan (#9)	3 minutes	legs
3. Hands Palmed, Arms Straight (#13)	3 minutes	aura
4. Stand Back to Back (#21)	3 minutes	aura
5. Hand to Heart (#22)	3 minutes	heart center
6. Third Eyes Touching (#24)	3 minutes	third eye
7. Meditate Face to Face (#27)	10 minutes	
	Total: 28 minutes	

Example of an expanded set

Table 2b.

	Time	Area Affected
1. Seesaw (#10)	3 minutes	spine
2. Squats (#7)	3 minutes	legs
3. Tricuti Kriya (#12V)	3 minutes	aura balance
4. Arms Up 60° (#15)	3 minutes	upper aura
5. Legs Up outside Arms (#17V)	3 minutes	lower aura
6. Fingerlock at Heart (#18)	3 minutes	middle aura
7. Arica Breath Coordination (#19)	5 minutes	
8. Heart Beam (#25)	10 minutes	heart center
9. Third Eye Beam (#26)	3 minutes	third eye
10. Crown Centers Touching (#23)	3 minutes	crown center
11. Meditate with Mantra (#29)	15 minutes	
	Total: 54 minutes	

Part II. The Exercises

Tantric Exercises

Before and After Practice

The traditional time for doing yoga is in the early morning, but any quiet time will do. Choose a time when neither partner has to rush off immediately afterwards, and a place where the chances of being disturbed are minimal (you might want to leave the phone off the hook). Do not eat for several hours beforehand, or else eat only very lightly.

Any bathing should be prior to the session. Traditional practitioners bathe immediately before yoga practice as a kind of preparatory ritual.

Always begin by relaxing and tuning in. Sit comfortably with a straight spine, close the eyes, and join the palms together in a "prayer pose" in front of the heart. The joints of the thumbs are pressed into the chest with a slight but definite pressure. This pose calms the mind by momentarily restricting some of the energy flows of the body and by applying pressure on the mind nerve (one of the nadis which directly influences the mental state), which is in the center of the chest.

Go within and feel that you are asking your own higher self, your own inner teacher, for guidance. Imagine that you are tuning into the intuitive source. (If you feel close to a specific teacher, then ask for her or his guidance and protection.) Remain in this attitude for 2–3 minutes, or until you feel "tuned in."

Next, become aware of your body. Imagine/feel that you are interpenetrated and surrounded by an energy field, and then imagine that your partner's energy body is touching yours. Finally, feel that the two fields are blending in such a way that energy currents are flowing back and forth between them. Only then should you open the eyes and begin.

At the completion of an exercise or a series of exercises, go through the same procedure in reverse. Close the eyes, and then gradually draw the energy back, allowing a very subtle but definite barrier to arise between you and your partner. This can be seen as a very loving barrier, rather than a heavy metal door. At the deepest level we are all really One, but at another level individuality has a definite purpose, which must be respected; thus the processes of opening and closing the energy field are crucial.

At the conclusion of a long meditative exercise, it is helpful to stretch the arms up and go through a cycle of inhaling and exhaling. Only after the stretching and breathing are completed should the legs be extended. If the meditation has continued a long time, the partners might massage each other's legs. (Squeeze fairly hard during this massage to promote circulation.) Partners might also exchange a back massage.

Basic Energy Awareness Techniques

Simple energy awareness exercises allow us to come in touch with the energy body; they help us to translate "energy" from a vague conception into a perceptible reality. For this reason energy awareness exercises are useful as preliminaries to the other tantric yoga techniques.

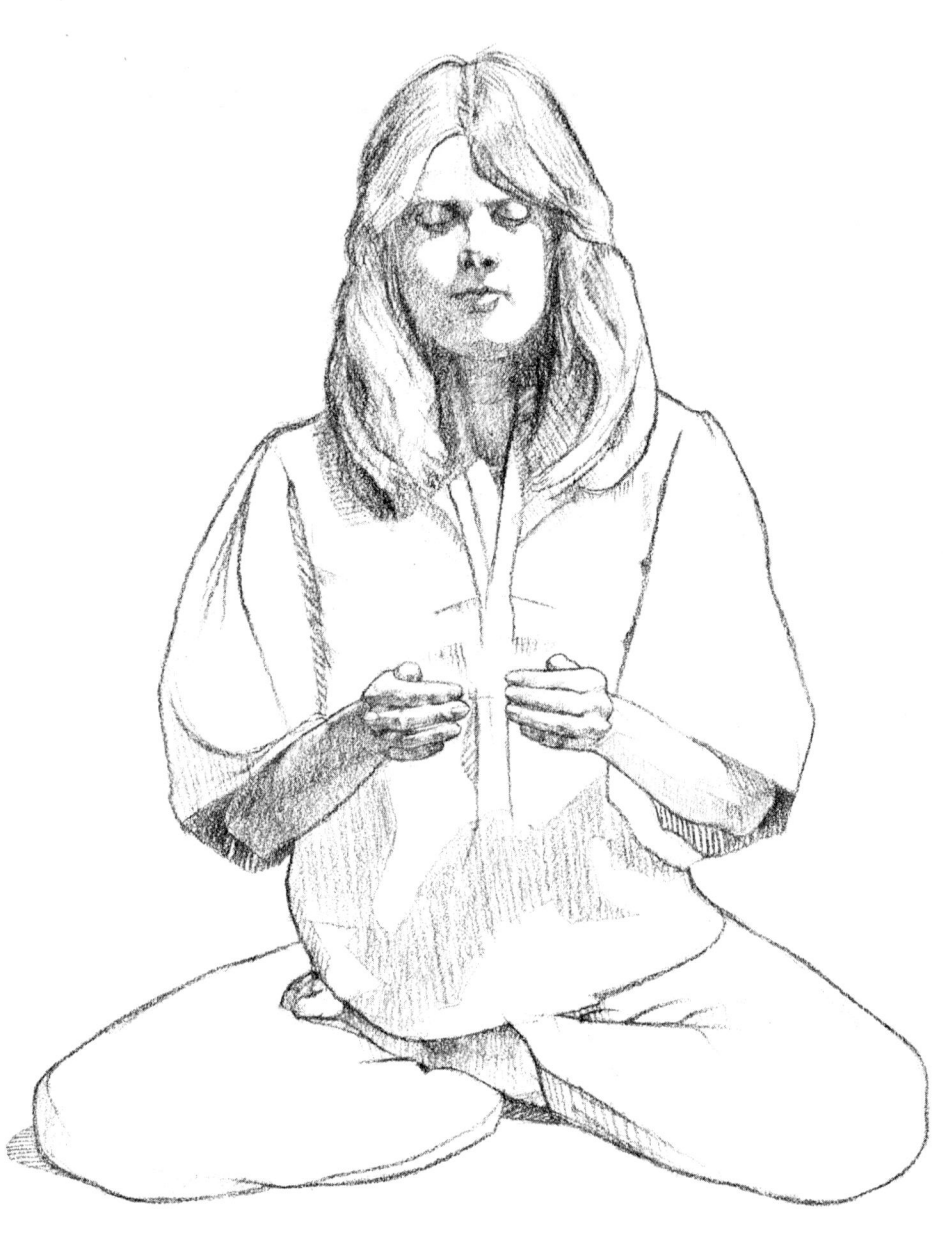

Preliminary Energy Awareness

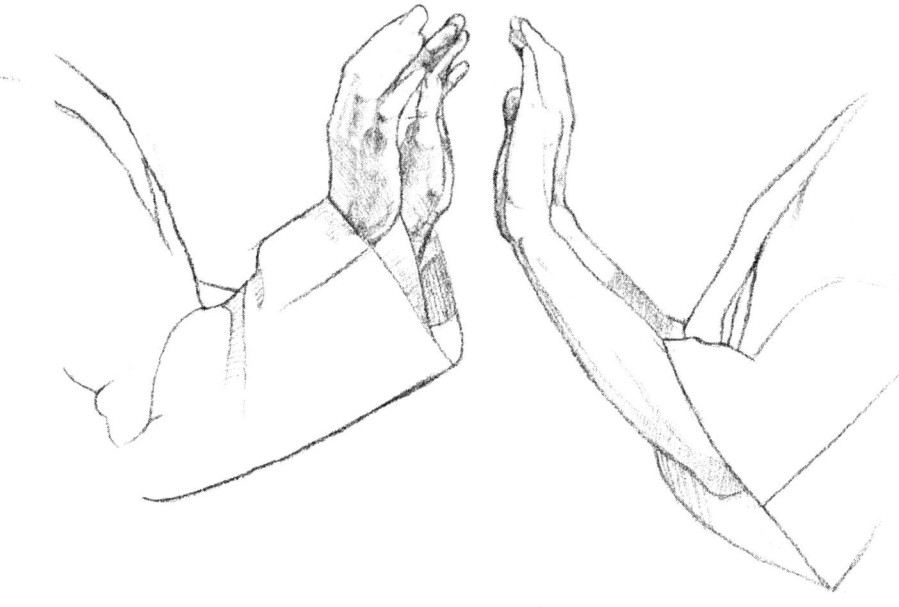

1. Magnetic Energy Awareness

Time: 2–3 minutes

If you have never worked with these techniques before, or if you are introducing them to someone else for the first time, begin with a simple energy awareness experiment. Bring your palms close together but not touching. Then move your hands very slowly in small circles or back and forth slightly. Remain as relaxed as possible. In a few minutes a distinct magnetic feeling will develop.

Now concentrate on creating the magnetic energy feeling between your palms and the palms of the partner. Raise the hands to almost shoulder level, and bring palms within an inch or two of the partner's palms. Try to avoid contact with the partner's hands. Move the hands *slightly* and *slowly* in various directions.

As you play with this technique, focus on feeling the energy rather than on becoming involved in intense eye contact.

2. Energy Flow through Fingertips   Time: 3–5 minutes

Sitting on the heels, partners touch knees. The hands are then extended out at shoulder level, until the partners are touching each other's finger and thumb tips.

Put most of the concentration into the fingertips. Imagine that energy is flowing between you, and mentally try to create a feeling of "tingling" in the fingertips. Breathe normally. Eyes may be opened or closed.

Variation: Energy Flow through Palms
The same exercise may be done with the hands palmed.

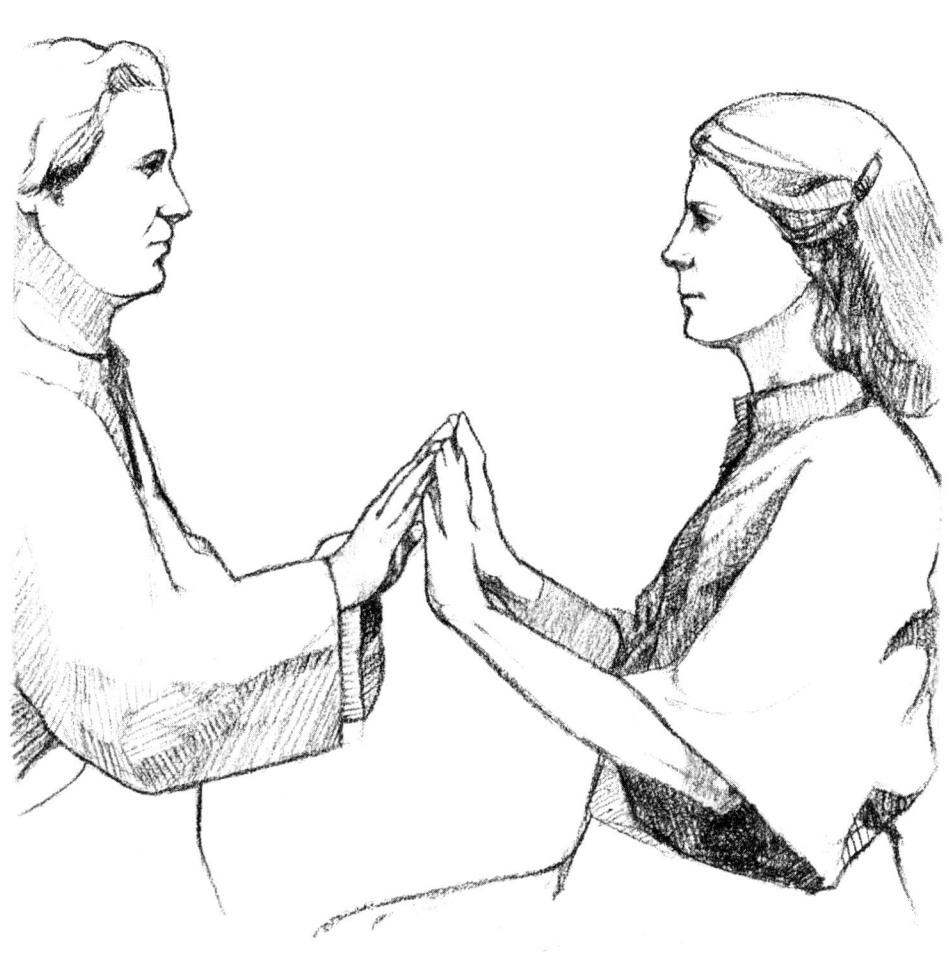

3. Energy Flow through Saturn Fingers Time: 3–5 minutes

Lie down on the stomach. Arch the upper part of the body up, supported by the elbows. Forearms are on the floor with the palms together; the longest fingers touch the tips of the partner's longest fingers. Feel energy flow across the point of contact.

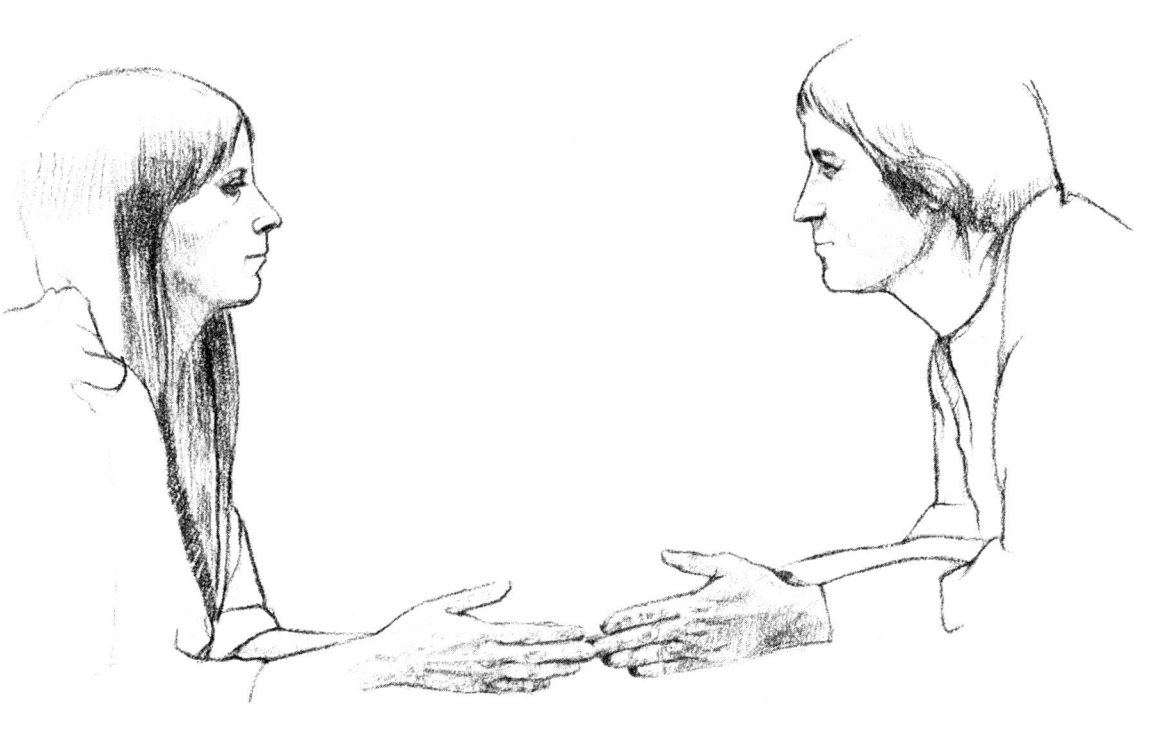

4. Energy Flow through Soles, Sitting Up   Time: 3–5 minutes

With straight legs, sit so that the soles of the feet are joined flat with the partner's. The hands may rest on the legs, or else they may be brought back to prop up the body. Feel the energy flow in the soles of the feet.

Variation: Energy Flow through Soles, Lying Down
    Lie down on the back with the feet joined.

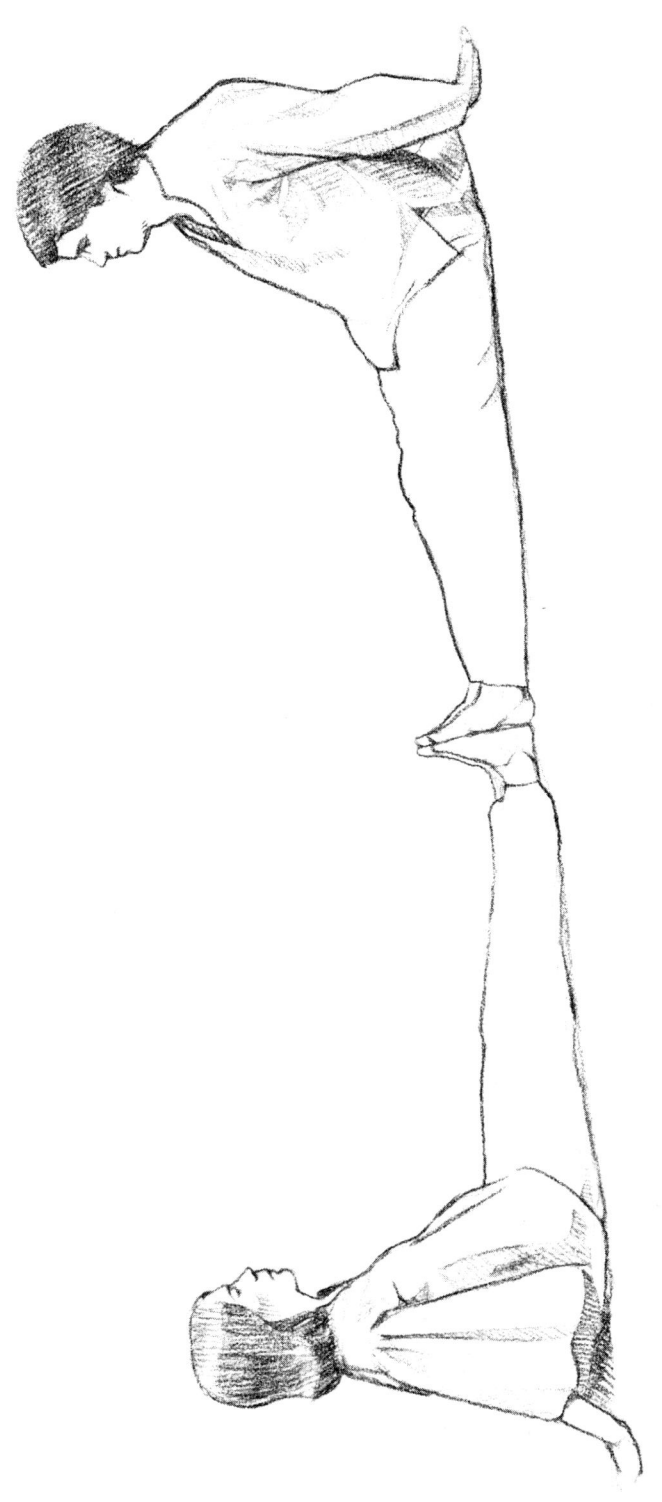

5. Hold Shoulder

Time: 3–5 minutes

Sit on the heels, with knees touching partner's knees. Bring the arms out so that partners are holding each other's shoulders. Try to become aware of energy flowing along the arms and the hands.

Since this position produces an intrusion on each individual's personal space, thus bringing psychological defense mechanisms to the surface, there is a special need to relax consciously during this pose.

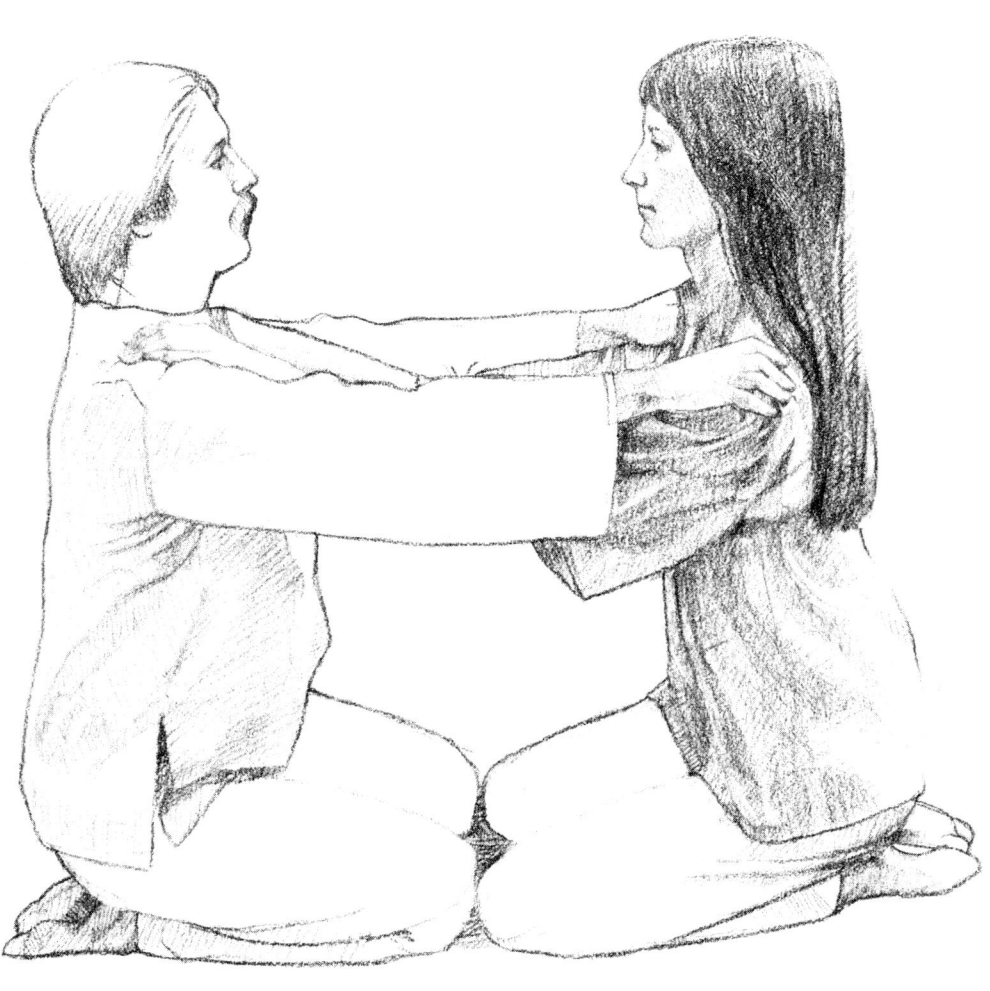

Tantric Yoga Exercises

The exercises in this section have the purpose of preparing the physical body for longer, deeper techniques, by promoting spinal flexibility and stimulating circulation.

6. Spinal Flex, Legs Crossed

Time: 3–5 minutes*

Sit cross-legged and hold the legs where they cross. Facing the partner, with the gaze joined, begin a spinal flex: inhale flexing forward, and exhale flexing back, keeping the head level enough to maintain eye contact. Partners should coordinate the movements.

This exercise may be done slowly, with deep breathing, or rapidly, with powerful breathing. When the exercise is done slowly, the rate of speed of the flexing should be determined by the partner with the smallest lung capacity. (In other words, the length of time that it takes for that person to inhale and exhale a comfortable deep breath should be the length of time of the complete movement.) When done rapidly, the rate of speed of the flexing should be about one complete movement per second.

At the end of the exercise, bring the back erect. Inhale, exhale, inhale, and hold briefly. Then gently exhale and relax.

Variation: Spinal Flex on Heels
   Do this exercise sitting on or between the heels.

*Note: If you start to feel faint stop sooner, or breath more shallowly (a faint feeling may indicate that the breaths have been too deep).

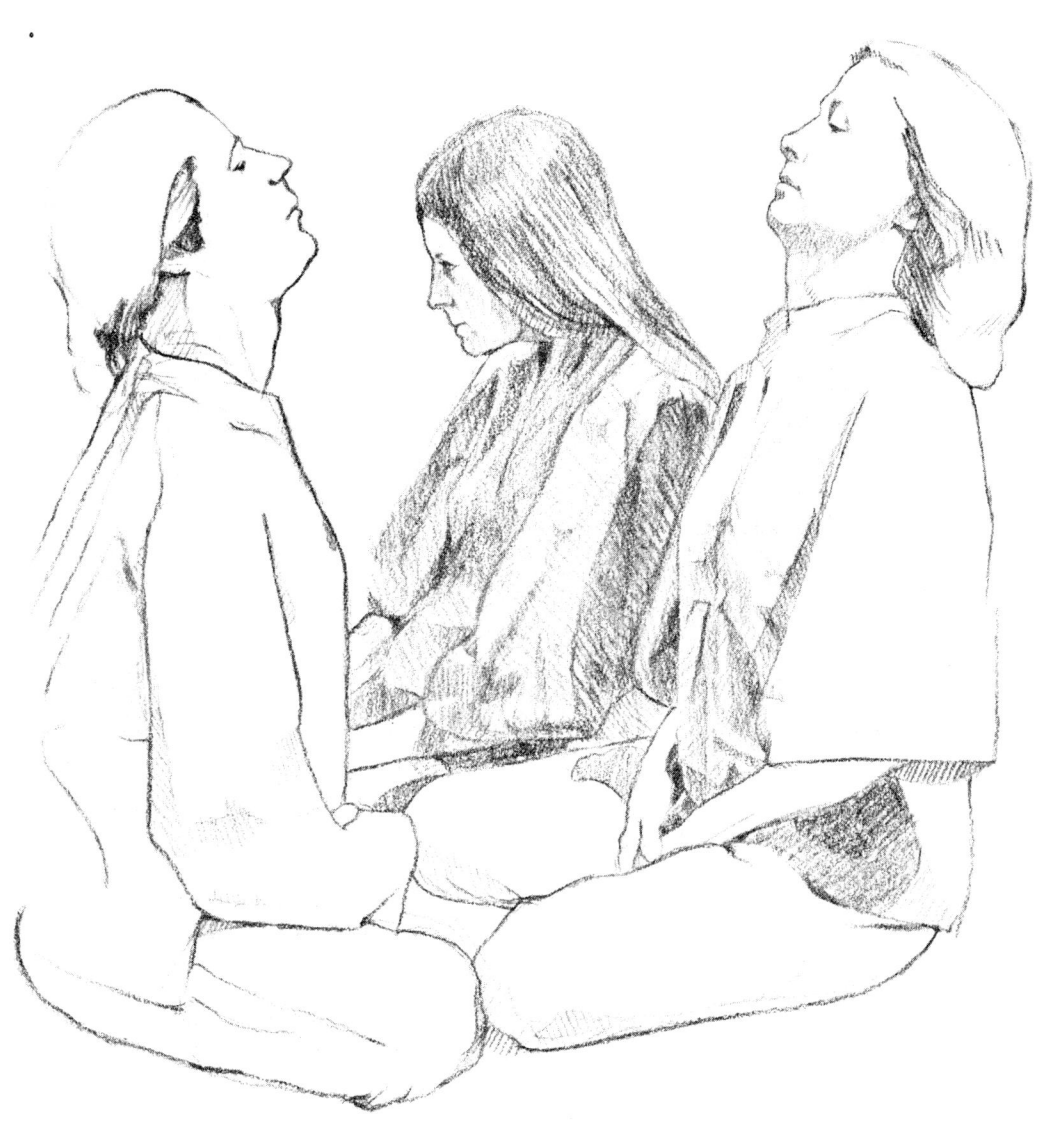

7. Squats

Time: 3–5 minutes*

Stand with the hands holding the partner's hands (fingers interlocked). With long, deep breaths, exhale squatting down, inhale standing up; continue thus, up and down. The length of time of each movement should be the length of a comfortable deep breath.

At the end of the exercise, squat down, inhale, and hold the breath in for a moment (10–15 seconds); then exhale, relax, and breath normally.

Variation: Rise up on the toes during the pause between inhalation and exhalation.

* Note: If you start to feel faint, stop immediately, sit down, and breathe normally.

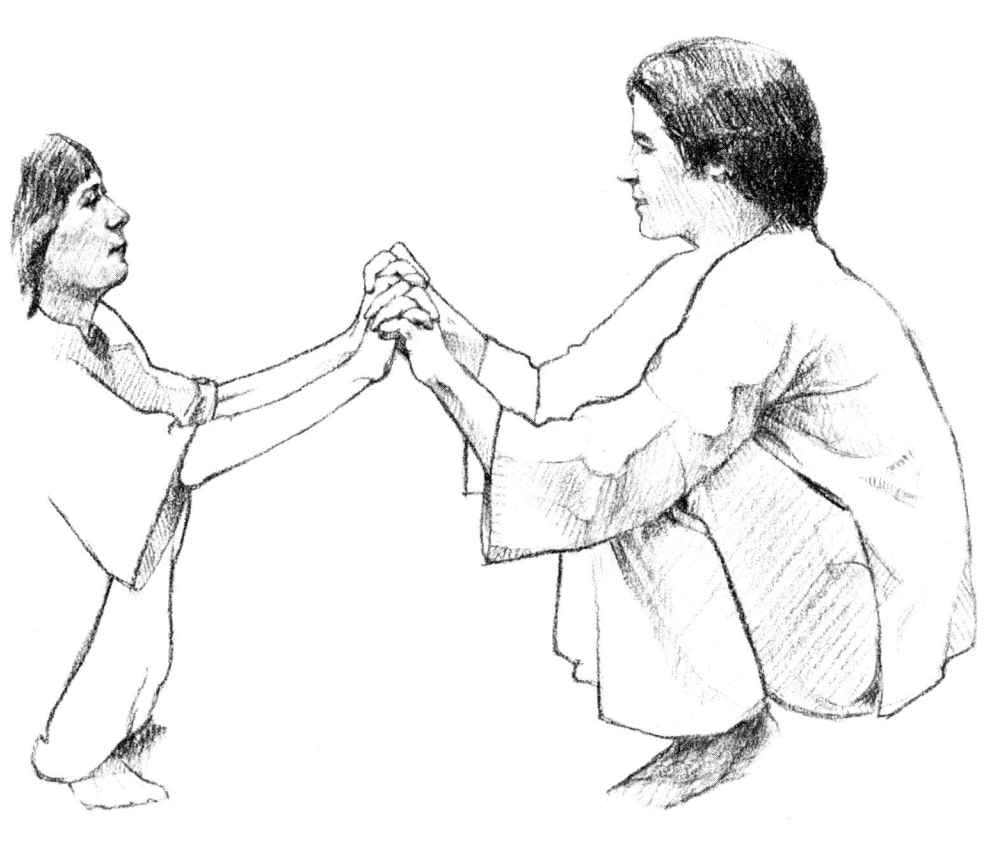

8. Crow Pose

Time: 3–5 minutes

Squat down until the knees touch the chest. Join hands with the partner. Hold the posture and do long, deep breathing or short, rapid breathing.

At the end of the exercise, inhale, exhale, inhale and hold for a moment (10–15 seconds); then exhale, breathe normally, and relax.

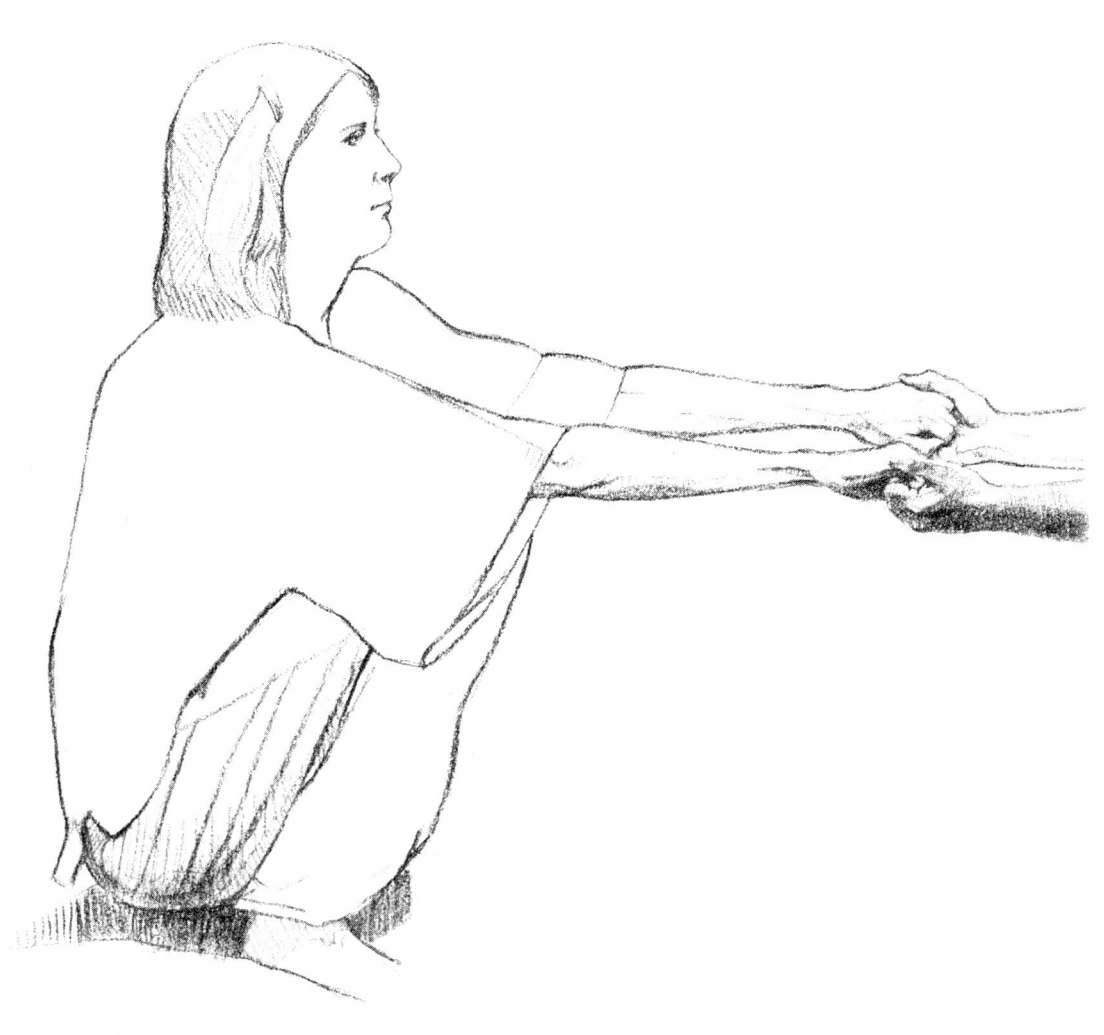

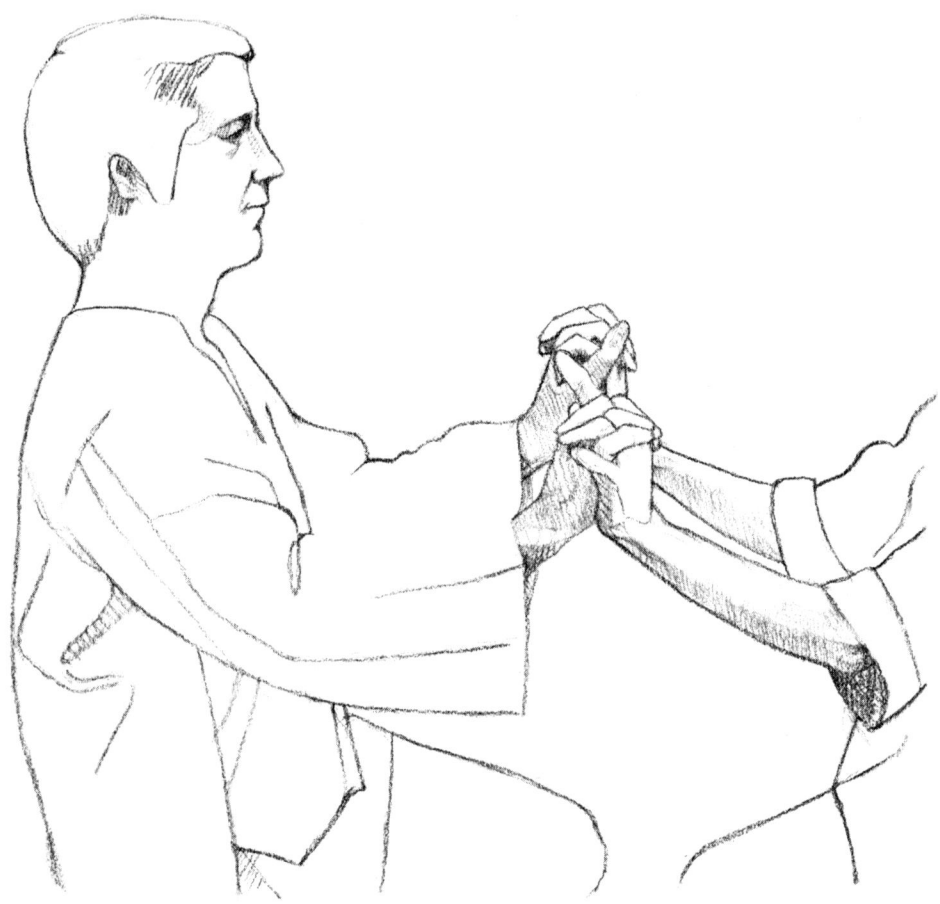

9. Rising Vajrasan

Time: 3–5 minutes

Sit on the heels with the knees close to (but not touching) the partner's knees. Interlock hands with the partner's hands at shoulder level. Inhale and rise up off of the heels until the body straightens (hands simultaneously rise up over the head). Then exhale, sitting back down. Continue this up-and-down movement. The length of time for each movement should be the length of a comfortable deep breath.

At the end of the exercise, sit down, inhale, exhale, inhale, and hold for a moment (10–15 seconds). Then slowly exhale, breathe normally, and relax.

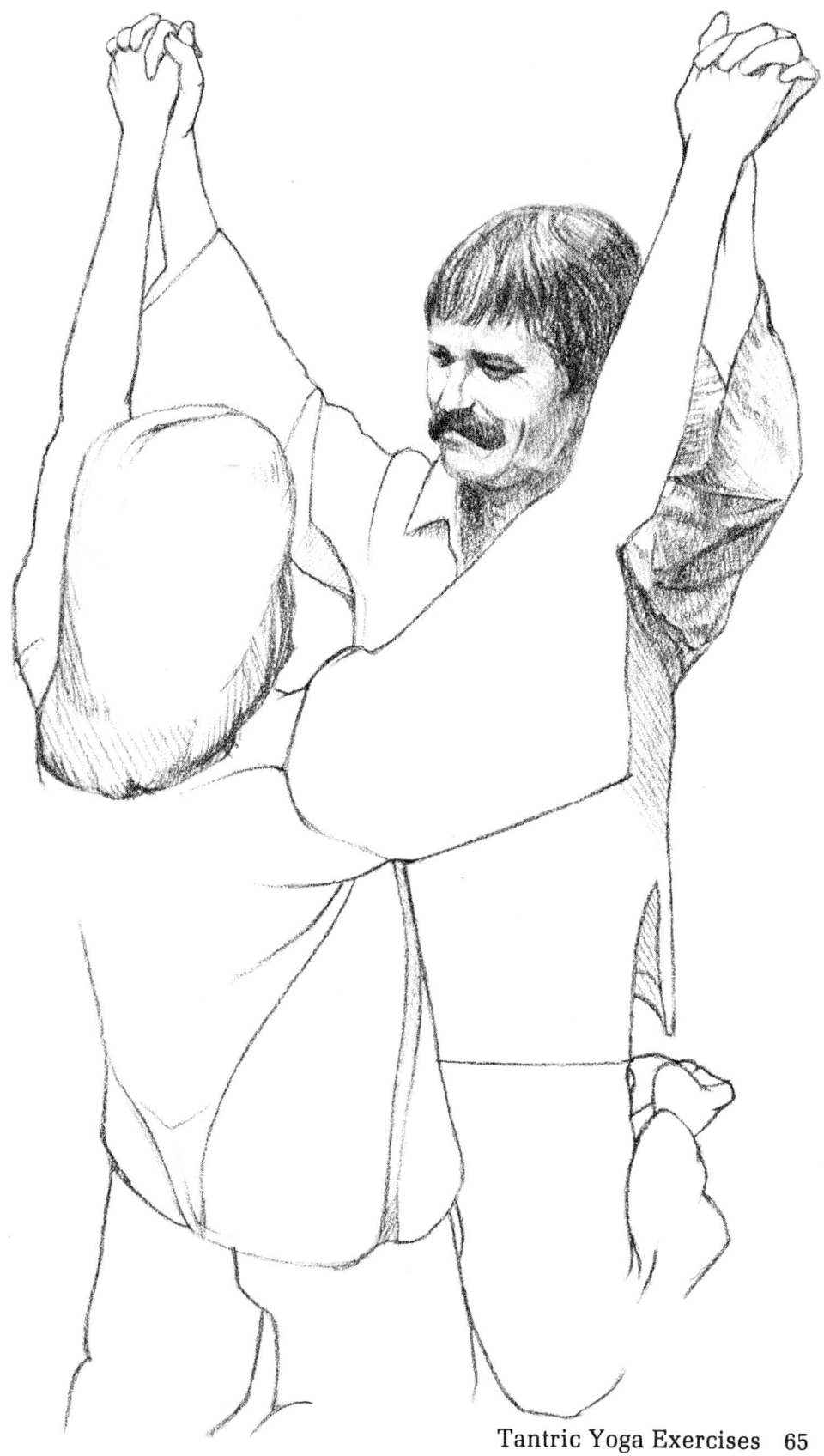

Tantric Yoga Exercises

## 10. Seesaw	Time: 3–5 minutes

Sit cross-legged or on the heels, with the knees touching the partner's knees. Clasp partner's hands or wrists. Inhaling, one person leans back, arching, until the top of the head touches the floor, while the partner supports him/her and leans forward, exhaling. Then the breaths change and the positions are gradually exchanged. The length of time for each movement should be the length of time for a comfortable deep breath.

At the end of the exercise, both partners sit up, inhale, exhale, inhale, and hold for a moment (10–15 seconds). Then slowly exhale, breathe normally, and relax.

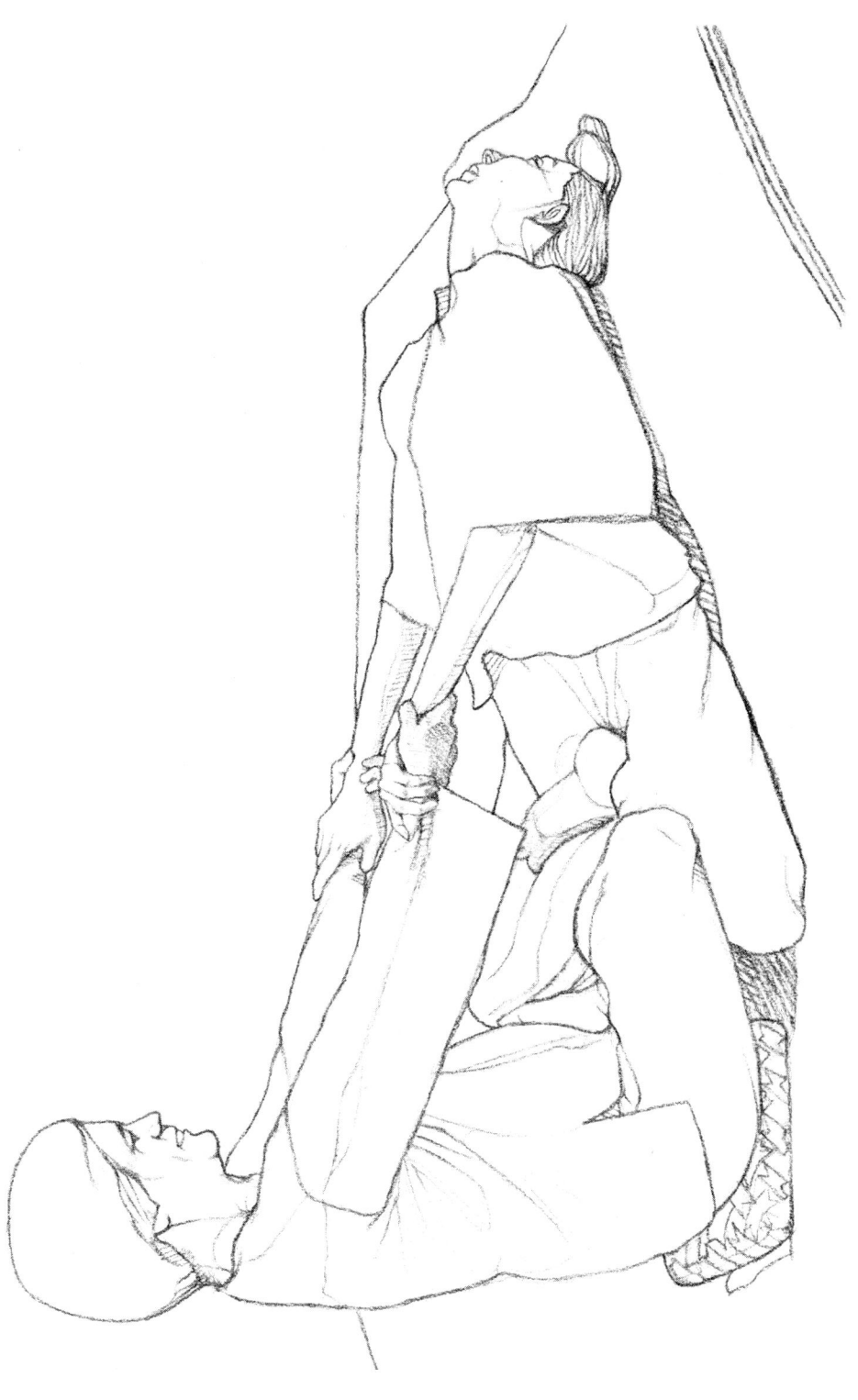

11. Moving Cobra Pose

Time: 3–5 minutes

Facing each other, lie down on the stomach with the head 6–12 inches away from the partner's head. Bring the hands underneath the shoulders, palms down; elbows and arms should be alongside the body rather than pointed out to the sides. Inhaling, straighten the arms up so that the body rises up (cobra pose). Exhaling, come back down. The length of time for one complete movement is the length of one comfortable deep breath.

At the end of the exercise, come up into the cobra pose, inhale, exhale, inhale, and hold the breath in for a moment (10–15 seconds). Then, slowly exhaling, come down, breathe normally, and relax.

Variation: Stationary Cobra Pose

Remain up in cobra pose and do long, deep breathing or short, rapid breathing.

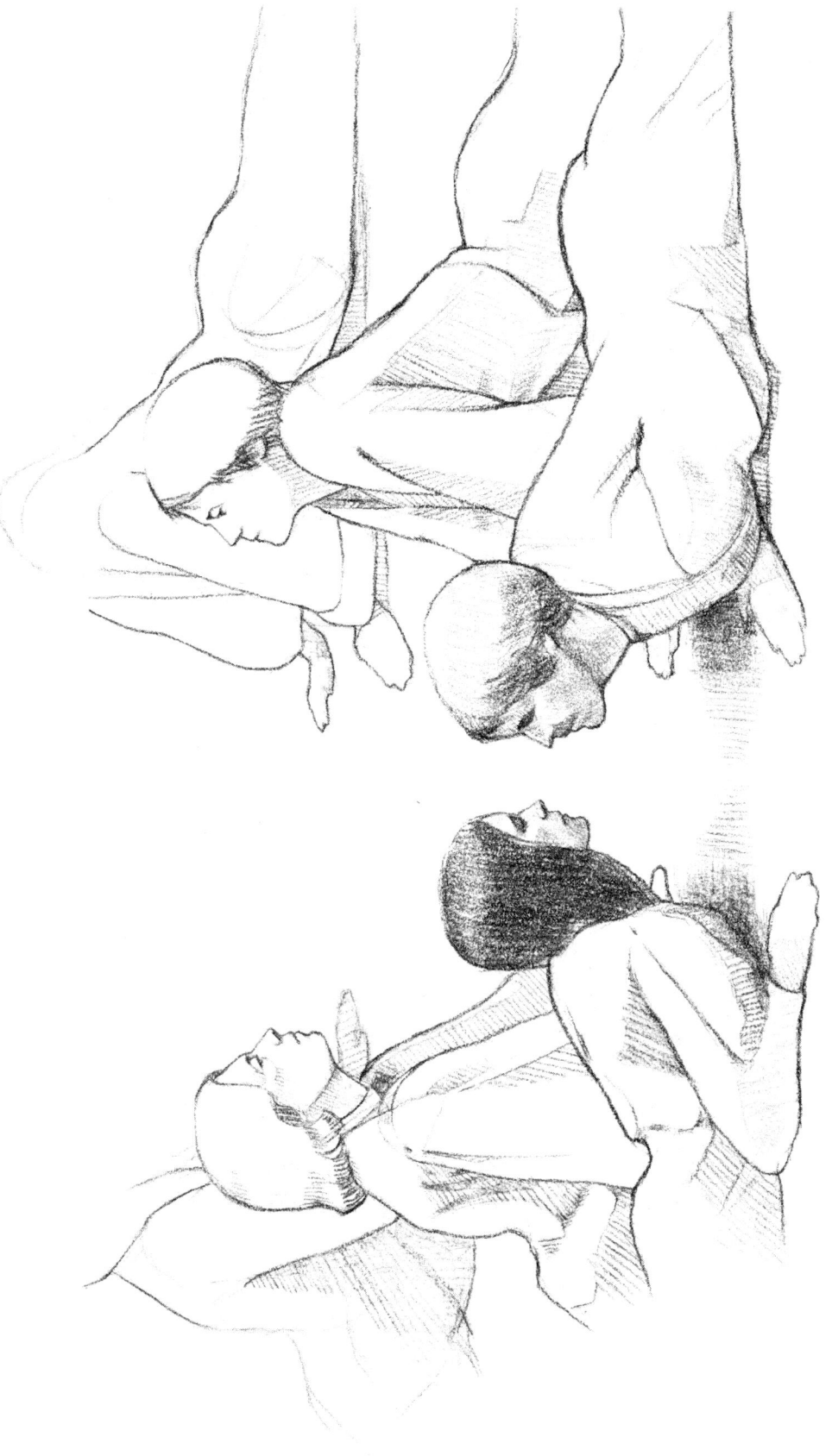

Magnetic Field Exercises

The exercises in this section are designed to affect the aura, that part of the subtle body which extends beyond the surface of the skin. During most of these techniques, the arms and/or the legs are extended and a powerful breath is used. This procedure channels the prana being taken in via the breath out through the limbs and into the energy field, so that the field becomes highly "charged."

Although the magnetic field exercises are highly physical, they prepare one for subtler techniques by energizing and clearing the energy channels. They are also good for blood circulation.

A minimal tantric yoga set would include at least one magnetic field exercise, but for those couples that have the time, four magnetic field exercises (done in any order) will produce a more complete "tune-up" of the aura:

1. An aura balancer (12 or 12V)
2. A technique which affects the lower part of the aura (17 or 17V)
3. A technique which affects the middle part of the aura (13, 14, or 18)
4. A technique which affects the upper part of the aura (15, 15V, 16, or 18)

In order to be really effective, the breath must be powerful—either short, rapid breathing or exaggerated long, deep breathing. Because it is difficult to do rapid breathing for very long, a good compromise is to begin with long, deep breathing and then change to short, rapid breathing halfway through the exercise. (People unaccustomed to such breathing may experience hyperventilation, and they should be careful to avoid fainting.) End each magnetic field exercise by inhaling, exhaling, inhaling, and holding the breath for a moment (10–15 seconds).

12. Tricuti Kriya, Rapid

Time: 3–5 minutes

Sit in any comfortable cross-legged pose facing the partner. Rest the hands in the lap in a venus lock (see p. 30). Coordinating movement with the partner, inhale slowly and deeply, leaning forward and to the right until the head touches the knee (either your own knee or partner's knee). Turn the head to the side as you bend forward, so that the gaze is not broken. Then begin exhaling, while straightening up and leaning forward and to the left, still not breaking the gaze, until the head touches the knee. Begin inhalation back up and continue the same movement. The movements should be smooth and continuous; do not pause in the upright position, and avoid the tendency to speed up.

The *tricuti* ("triangle") kriya evens out the charge density in the aura. (A balanced aura is important, because an imbalanced field will not hold a charge as well as an equally distributed field.) This exercise also works to balance the energy distribution between the upper and lower parts of the body, and between the right and left sides.

The effectiveness of this technique may be enhanced by mentally chanting the energy-balancing mantra "*Sat Nam*" ("True Name")—"Sat" on the inhale and "Nam" on the exhale.

Variation: Tricuti Kriya, Slow
    Exactly the same except inhale while bringing the body up and exhale while bringing the body down to each knee.

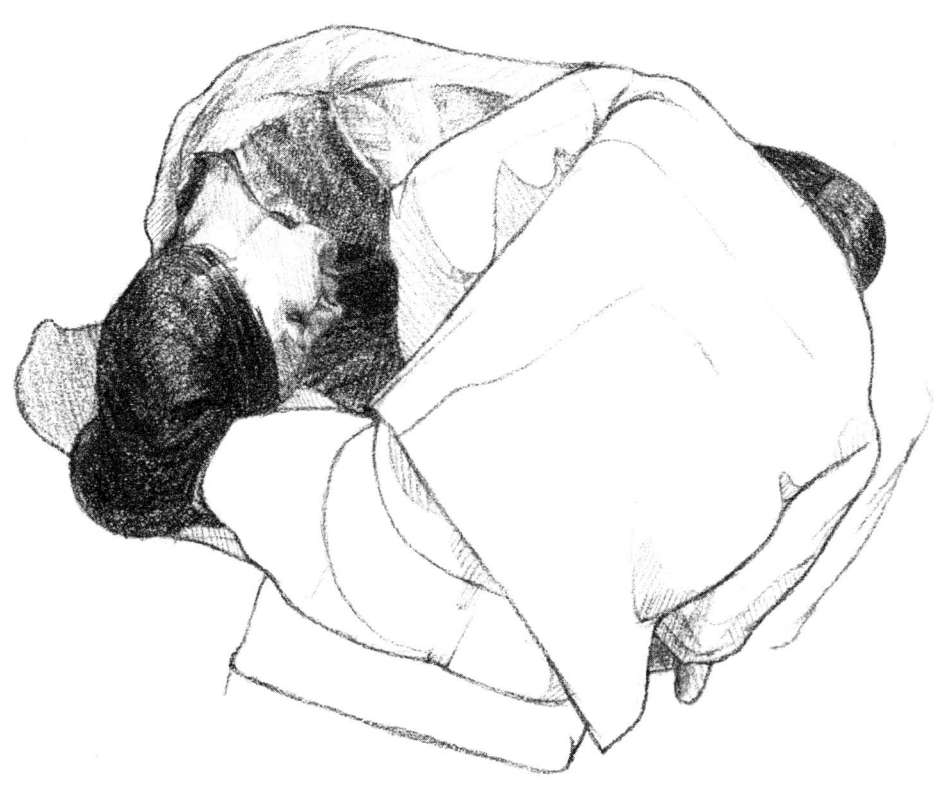

13. Hands Palmed, Arms Straight

Time: 3–5 minutes

Sit on the heels (knees not touching partner's knees), with the arms straight, palms pressed to those of the partner. Practice short, rapid breathing (preferably) or long, deep breathing.

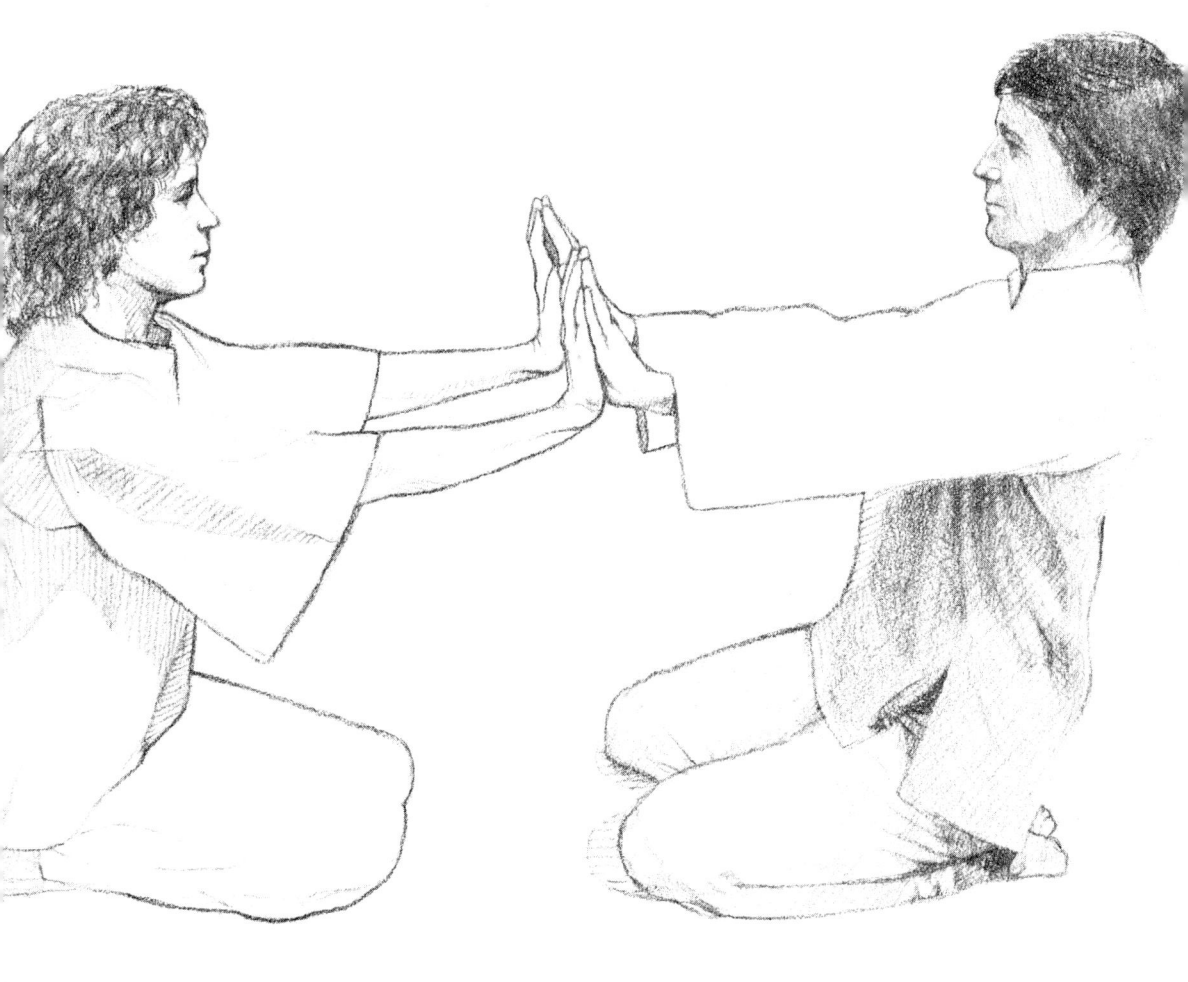

14. Hands Clasped, Lean Back Time: 3–5 minutes

Sit on the heels with knees touching partner's; clasping hands, both partners lean back as far as possible. Practice short, rapid breathing or long, deep breathing.

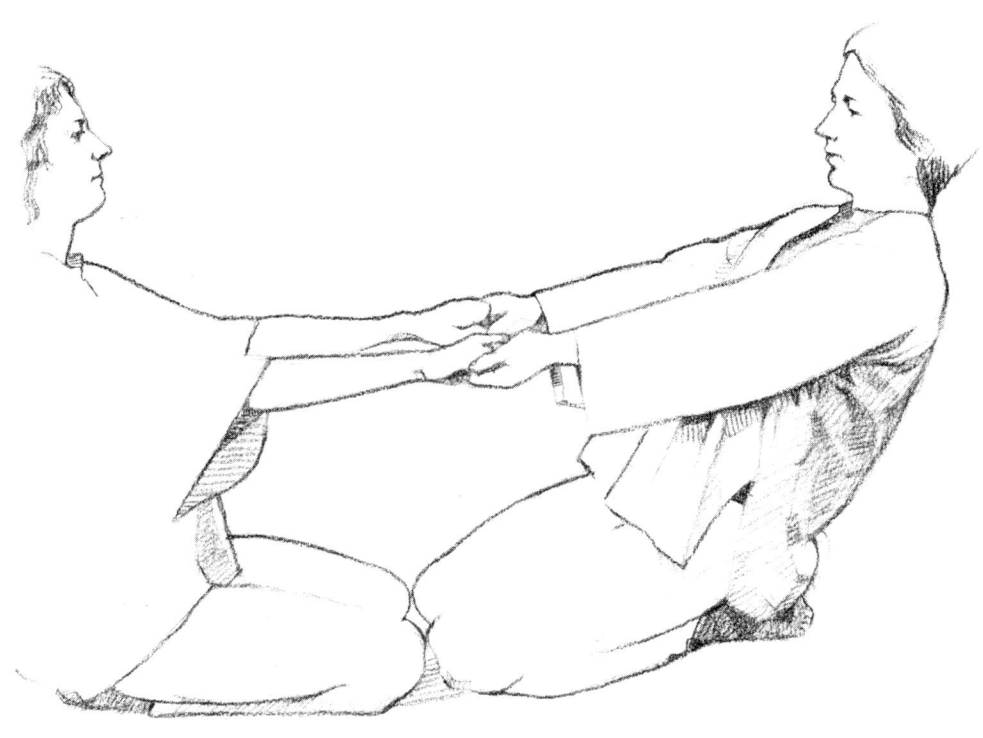

15. Arms Up 60 Degrees

Time: 3–5 minutes

Facing the partner, sit cross-legged or on the heels, with the knees touching. Bring the arms out to the sides and hold them, straight, at a 60-degree angle to the floor. Face the palms toward the partner's hands and hold them within a few inches of the partner's. Finally, spread the fingers so that a slight but definite tension is created in the palms. This will cause the prana to flow to the hands and charge up the aura around the hands. Practice long, deep breathing or short, rapid breathing.

Variation: Arms up 90 Degrees
   Keep the upper arms parallel to the ground, with elbows bent and hands stretched upward.

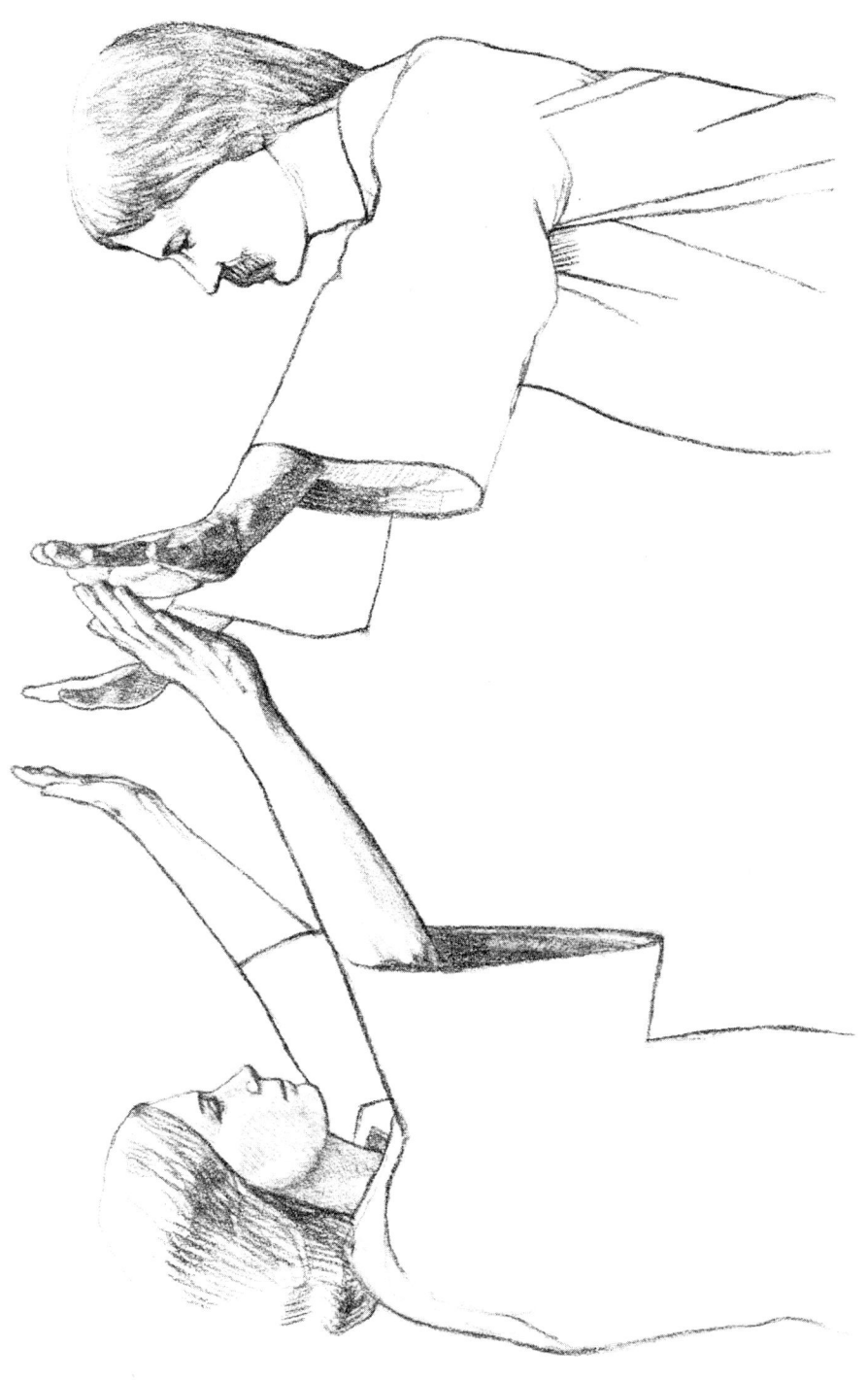

Magnetic Field Exercises 79

16. Back to Back, Arms Up 60 Degrees Time: 3–5 minutes

Sit cross-legged back to back so that the backs touch, but do not lean on each other. Bring arms out to the sides, making a 60-degree angle to the floor. Forearms touch and cross the partner's forearms so that the hands clasp. Practice long, deep breathing (preferably) or short, rapid breathing.

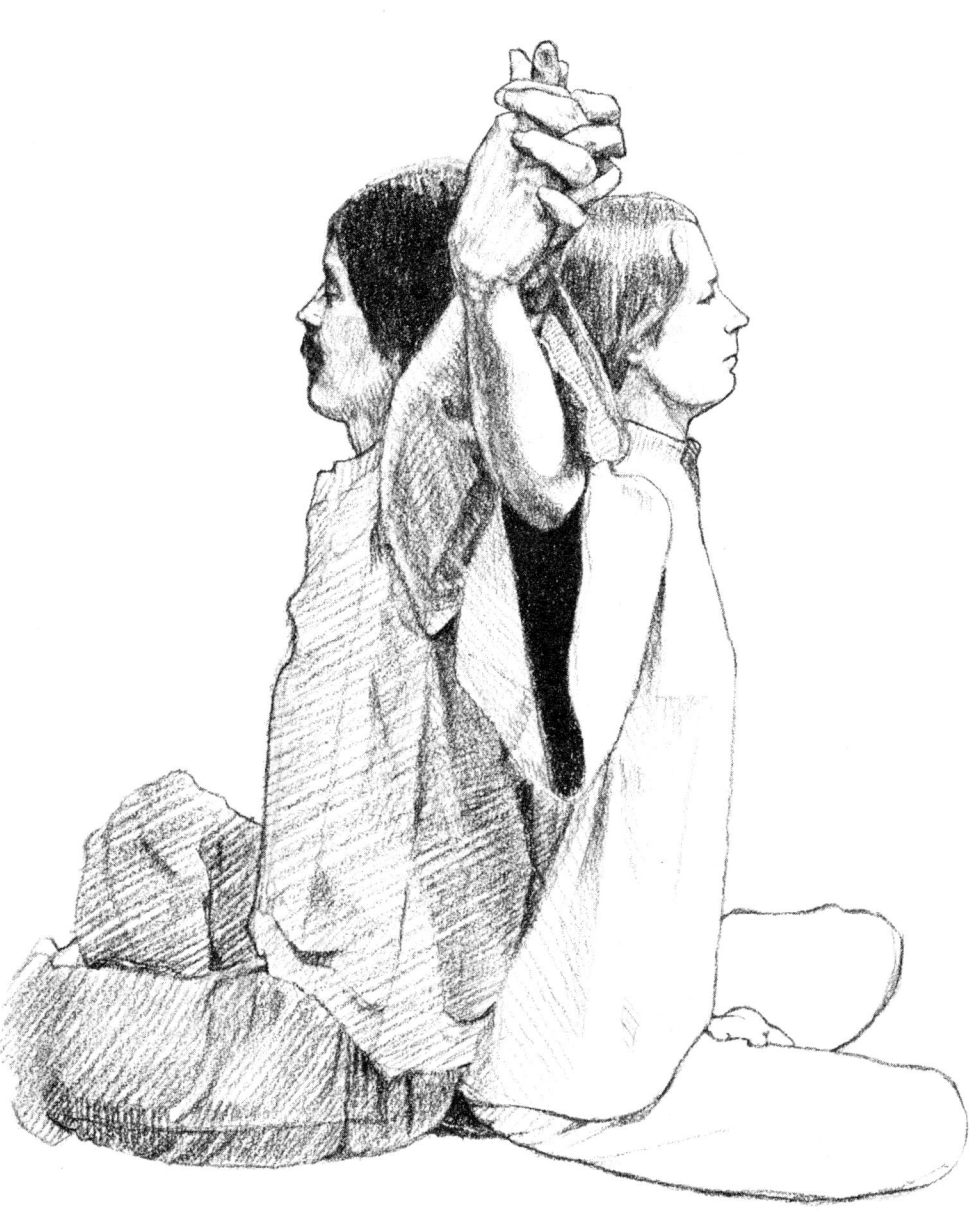

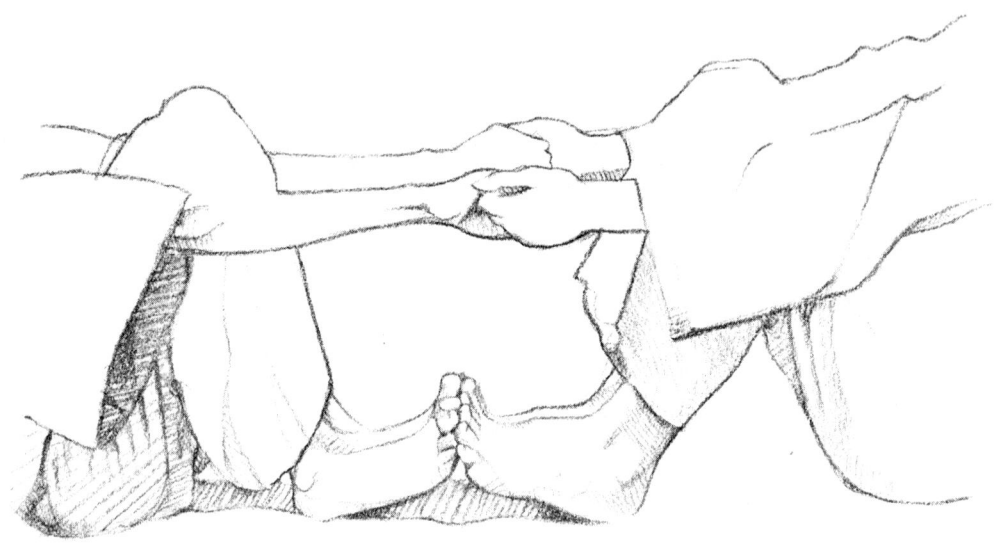

17. Legs Up inside Arms
Time: 1–3 minutes

Place the legs out in front of the body, with the knees bent, soles touching partner's. Hands are clasped outside of the legs and hooked together with partner's. Straighten the legs upward until a triangle is formed. (This position is not as difficult as it sounds.) Holding the legs up, begin short, rapid breathing or long, deep breathing.

Variation: Legs Up outside Arms
  Straighten the legs up outside of the arms.

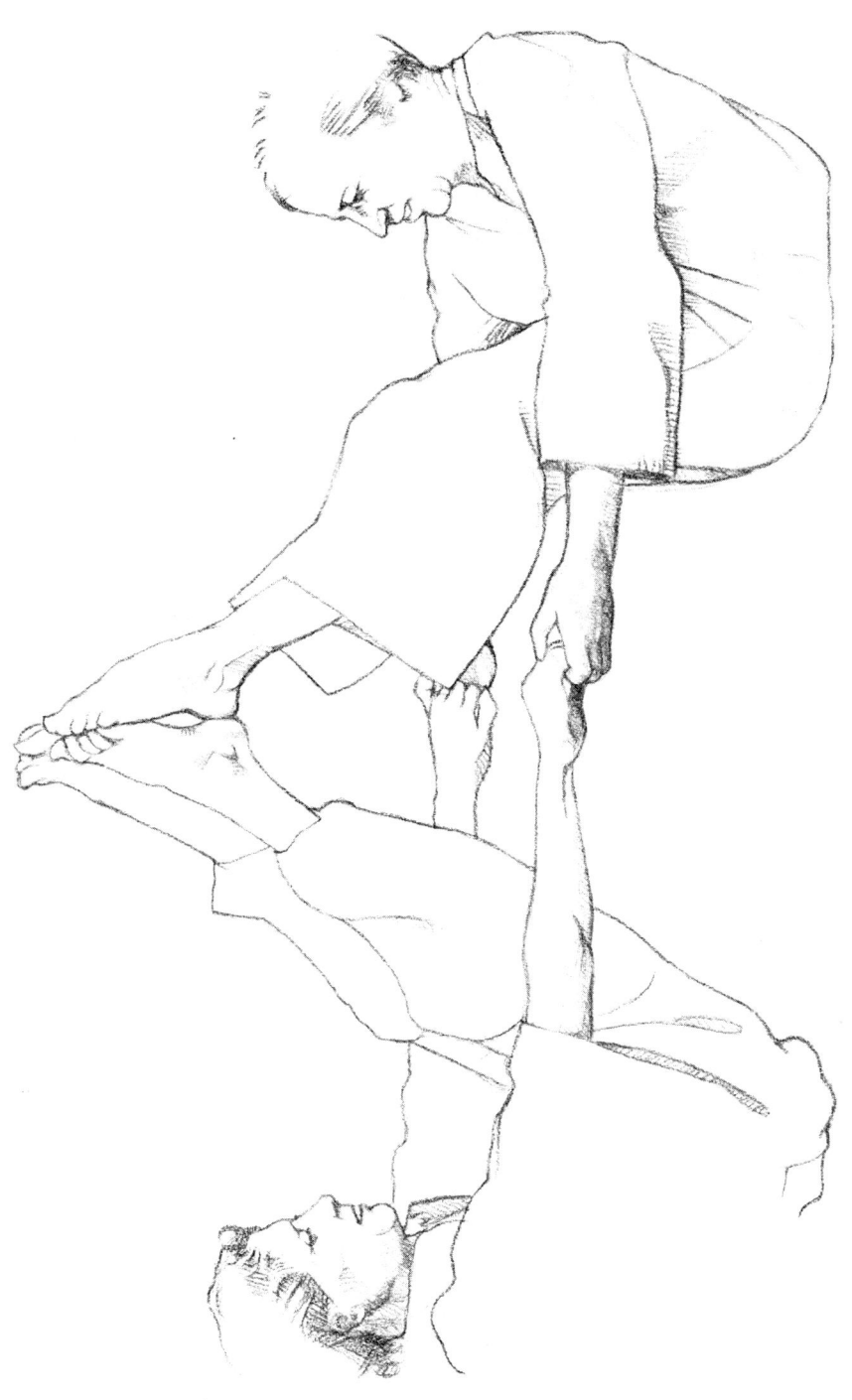

Magnetic Field Exercises 83

18. Finger Lock at Heart

Time: 3–5 minutes

Sitting cross-legged, hook the hands together in a finger lock in front of the heart (see p. 30). Keeping the hands an inch or so away from the surface of the chest, apply pressure as if trying to pull them apart. Focus the attention on the heart, and begin long, deep breathing or short, rapid breathing.

Variation: Finger Lock over Crown
   Hold the finger lock a few inches over the center of the top of the head.

Breath Coordination Techniques

The practices in this section tune a couple into each other by coordinating the breathing; simple physical movements or physical sensations guide the coordination. The simple action of coordinating the breath sets the major regulator of pranic energy (the breath) of both people on the same schedule, and thus enables the energy fields to blend together more easily and more deeply.

19. Arica Breath Coordination Time: 3-5 minutes

Facing the partner, sit on the heels or cross-legged, with the knees touching. Bring the arms out at about the level of the solar plexus, with one hand facing palm down and the other hand facing palm up. Bring the palms together with the partner's palms, or else hook the fingers together. Move one hand forward and the other hand back while inhaling. Then reverse the motion while exhaling. Continue the movement, synchronizing the breath. Avoid the tendency to speed up. This exercise will have a nice, dancing flow if both partners relax enough.

    The length of time for one complete movement is the length of one comfortable deep breath. End as the exercises in sections B and C were concluded, or simply pause, lower the hands, and breathe normally.

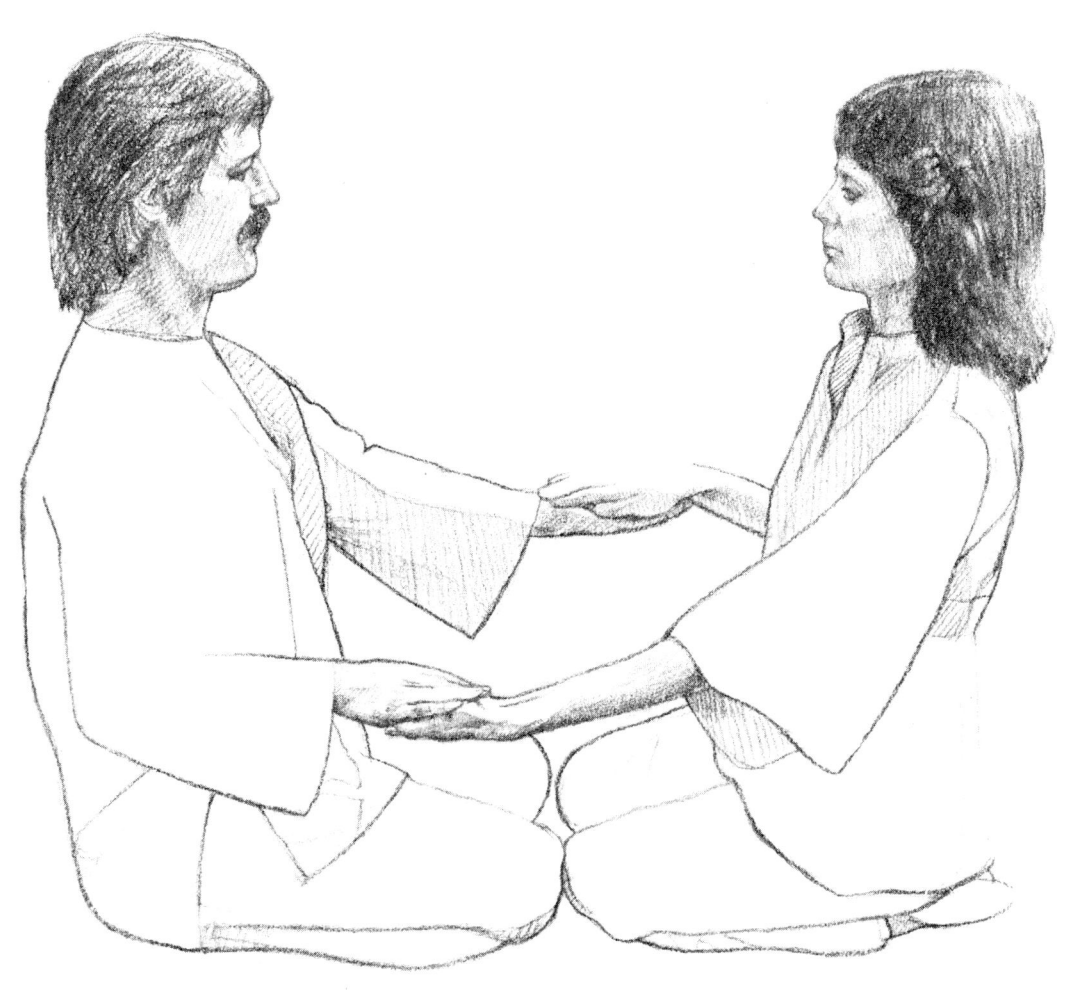

20. Finger-to-Knee Breath Coordination Time: 3–15 minutes

Sit on the heels or cross-legged, facing the partner. As one person begins exhaling, he or she lightly touches the partner's knee, who then inhales, so that one person is inhaling while the other person is exhaling. When the person who is inhaling completes the inhalation and begins exhaling, she or he then touches the partner's knee who stops exhaling and begins inhaling. This continues back and forth, so that first one person and then the other is guiding the breathing. The exercise may be done with moderate or relaxed deep breathing.

End by simply pausing and relaxing.

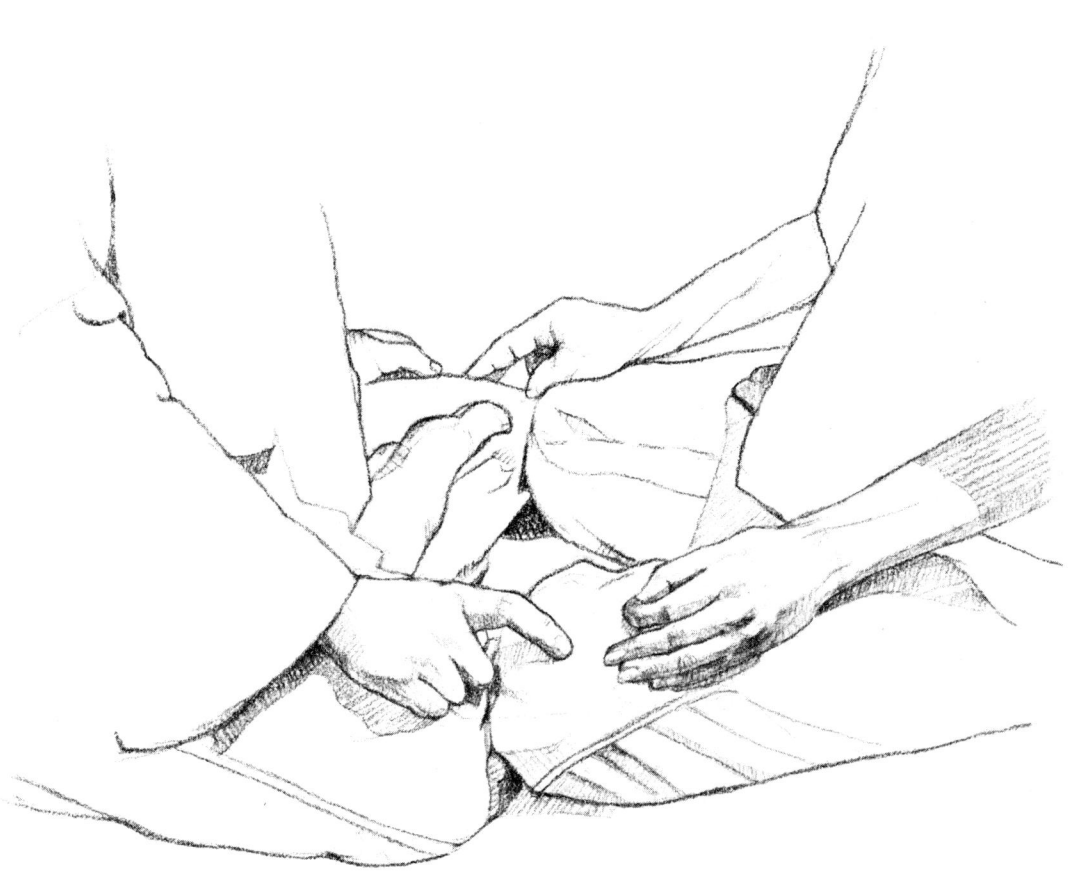

21. Stand Back to Back Time: 3–15 minutes

Partners stand back to back, with the hands clasped in a relaxed manner. Heads may touch, if there is not a great disparity in height. Coordinate the breathing so that both breathe together, or so that the breathing is reversed (one person exhales as the other inhales, and vice versa). Begin by having one partner lead the breathing while the other partner follows. Eventually try to breathe together with neither one leading. Use relaxed, long, deep breathing.

Meditate on the idea of being one soul in two bodies. Try to be sensitive to the subtle polarity change that the aura goes through as the "direction" of the breathing changes, from inhalation to exhalation or vice versa. Inhalation is yang (positive) and exhalation is yin (negative).

End by pausing, relaxing, and separating.

Variation: Sit Back to Back

Sit on the floor with the backs together. Legs may be crossed or extended.

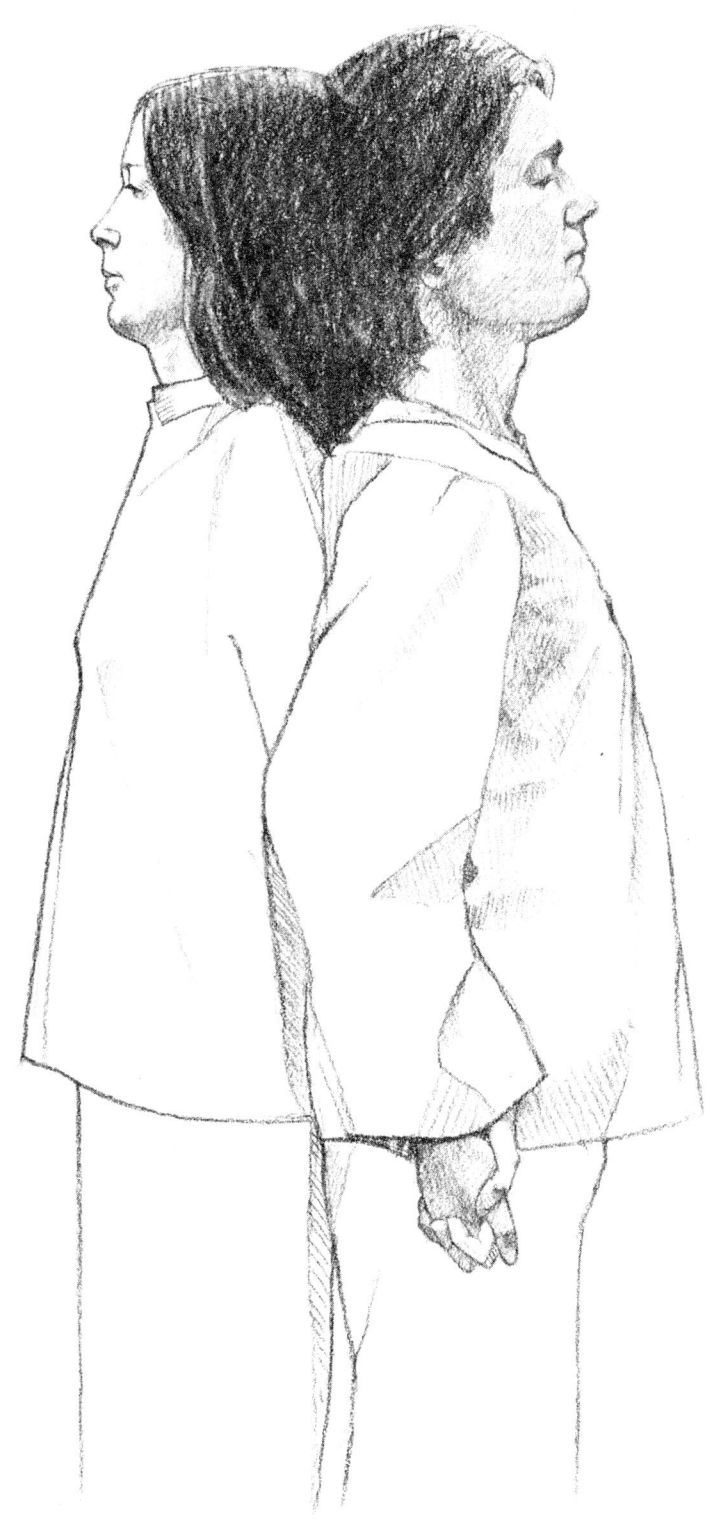

Subtle Awareness Exercises

The first set of energy awareness exercises (section A) utilized contact between the hands and the feet. The techniques in this section work with subtler energy flows between the chakras. Although the chakra energies may be difficult to perceive at first, the feeling of the current flows, once felt, are just as distinct.

Most of the exercises in this section work with the heart center and the brow center (the "third eye"); they are designed to break up emotional blocks and mental blocks, and to develop compassion and selfless love, as well as spiritual intuition and wisdom.

The usual approach to working with the chakras is to start with the lower centers and then move on to higher centers. When working with the techniques in this section, a heart center technique should be done first, then a brow center technique, then (if used) a crown center technique.

22. Hand to Heart

Time: 3–5 minutes*

Sitting in a comfortable cross-legged pose, with the knees touching partner's, place the right palm on the partner's chest, at the heart center. Bring the left hand up so that it covers the partner's right hand as if holding it to the heart. Imagine that you are inhaling Divine Love. Exhaling, project this energy out the arm and into the partner's heart. Focus on opening the partner's heart.

End by slowing down the energy flow, gently separating, and slowly lowering the arms.

* Note: The heart center technique can be built up to 10–15 minutes.

Variation: Finger to Third Eye

Apply the tip of the right index finger to the partner's third eye (between and slightly above the eyebrows). Join left hands in the lap, or else hold the palm of the left hand to your heart center. On the inhale, imagine that you are drawing in all of the knowledge and wisdom of the universe. On the exhale, visualize the energy flowing through your arm and into your partner's forehead. Focus on trying to open the partner's third eye.

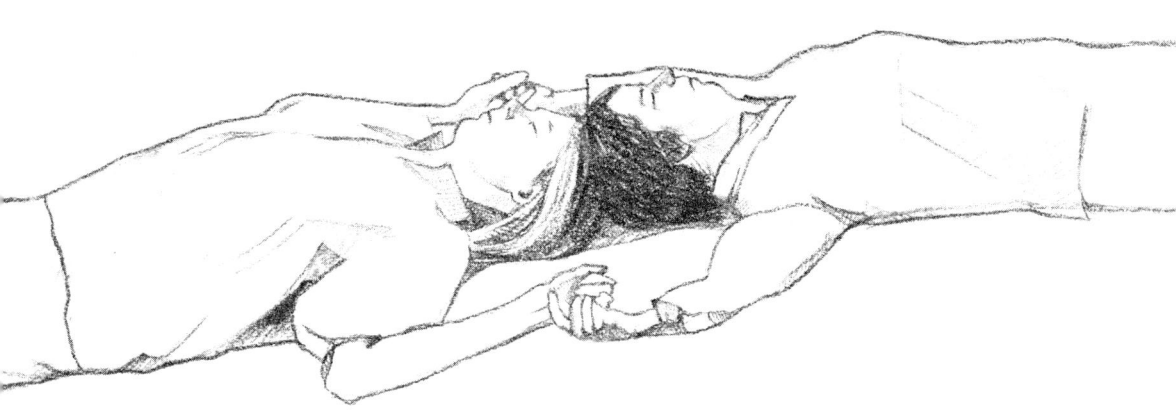

23. Crown Centers Touching

Time: 3–15 minutes

Lie down on the back, with the tops of the heads touching. Arms may be relaxed alongside the body or extended outward so that the partners can hold hands. Concentrate on the crown chakra, mentally producing a feeling of warmth and tingling where the partner's chakras join.

End by slowing down the energy flow and sitting up.

Variation: Crown Centers Apart

With heads separated by 6–12 inches, concentrate on projecting energy between the crown chakras. Visualize a beam of white or golden light.

24. Third Eyes Touching   Time: 3–15 minutes

Lying down on the side, join foreheads. Concentrate on sending energy back and forth between the third eyes.

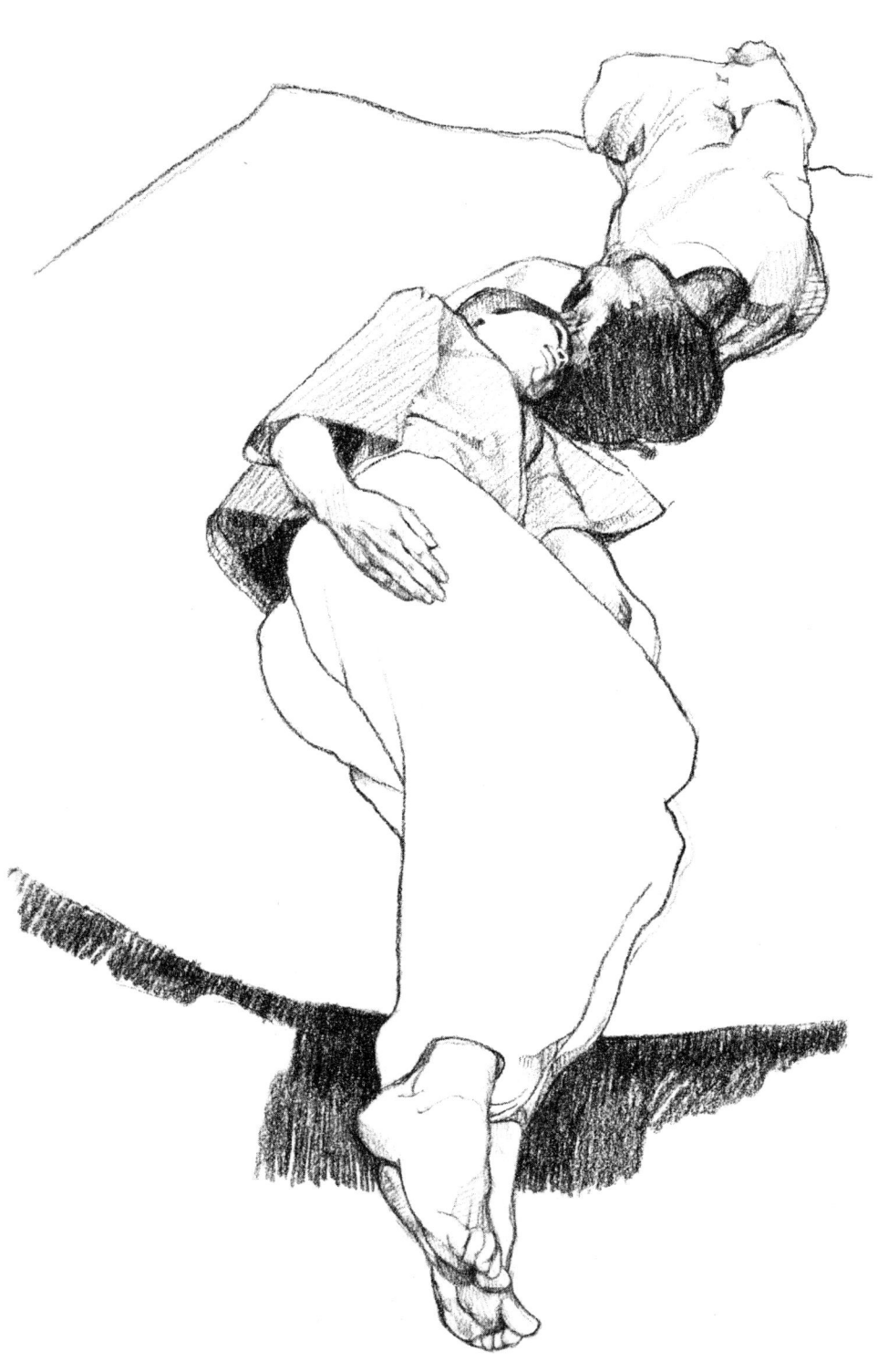

25. Heart Beam
Time: 5–15 minutes

Sit in any relaxed position facing the partner. Concentrate on the heart. Imagine that a beam of pure white or golden light 2–3 inches in diameter is radiating out of your heart and into the partner's heart. Focus on opening up and radiating a strong beam of love. Concentrate especially on the surface of the chest, developing a warm/tingling sensation at the source of the beam.

Variation: Heart Beam, Gaze at Chest
   Gaze at the partner's chest (at the heart chakra).

Variation: Heart Beam, Visualization
   Close the eyes and concentrate on the visualization.

Variation: Heart Beam, with Coordinated Breathing
   Coordinate the breaths in reverse, using the knee-touching technique described in exercise 20. The person exhaling projects energy, the person inhaling receives energy.

26. Third Eye Beam
Time: 3–15 minutes

Sit in any relaxed position facing the partner. Concentrate on the third eye. Imagine a beam of energy ½ inch in diameter radiating out of your third eye and into the partner's third eye. Focus on radiating intuitive wisdom.

Variation: Third Eye Beam, Visualization
   Close the eyes and concentrate on the visualization.

Variation: Third Eye Beam, Gaze at Forehead
   Fix the gaze on the partner's third eye and feel that energy is flowing from the eyes, through the gaze, and into the partner's third eye. Feel that the eyes focus energy, and meditate on the partner's third eye.

Variation: Third Eye Beam, with Coordinated Breathing
   Coordinate the breath in reverse, as in exercise 20.

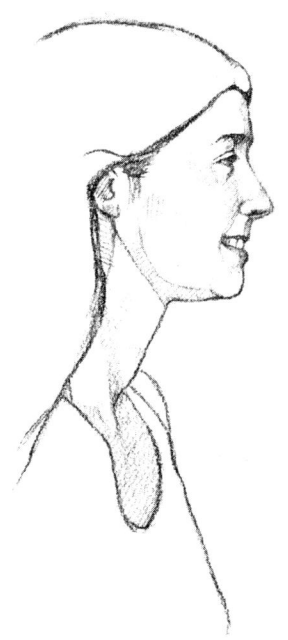
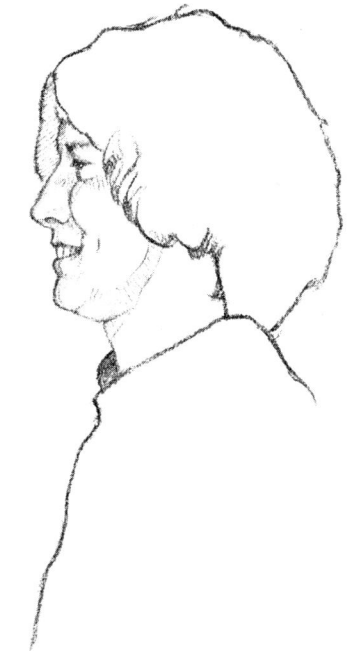

Tantric Meditations

The goal of the tantric meditation is cosmic consciousness, and union at the level of the soul.

27. Meditate Face to Face Time: 10–15 minutes

Sit facing the partner in any comfortable position. The hands should be held in a meditative mudra, such as the finger lock or venus lock (see page 30). Meditate steadily into the partner's eyes as if they were mandalas.

Variation: Meditate Holding Hands
   Hold the partner's hands in any relaxed way.

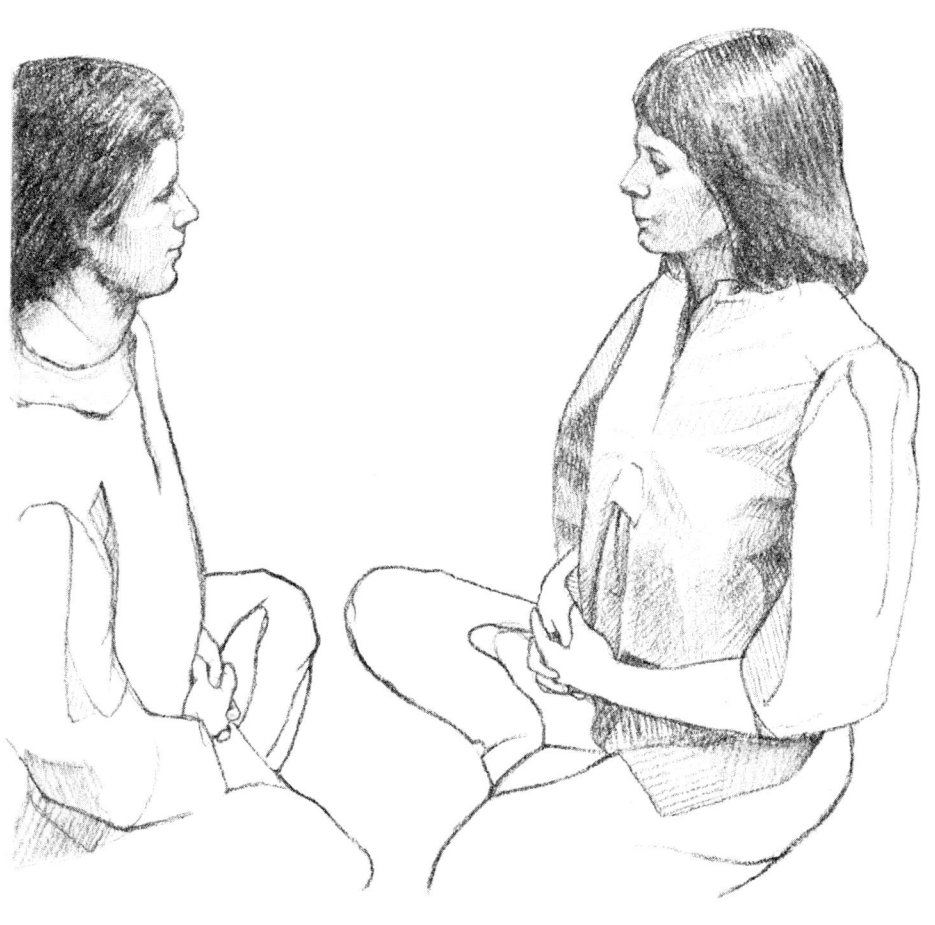

28. Meditate Back to Back   Time: Unlimited

Sit back to back, and meditate.

Variation: Spinal Heat
    Focus on moving energy up and down the spine, during inhalation and exhalation. Concentrate on feeling heat in the spine.

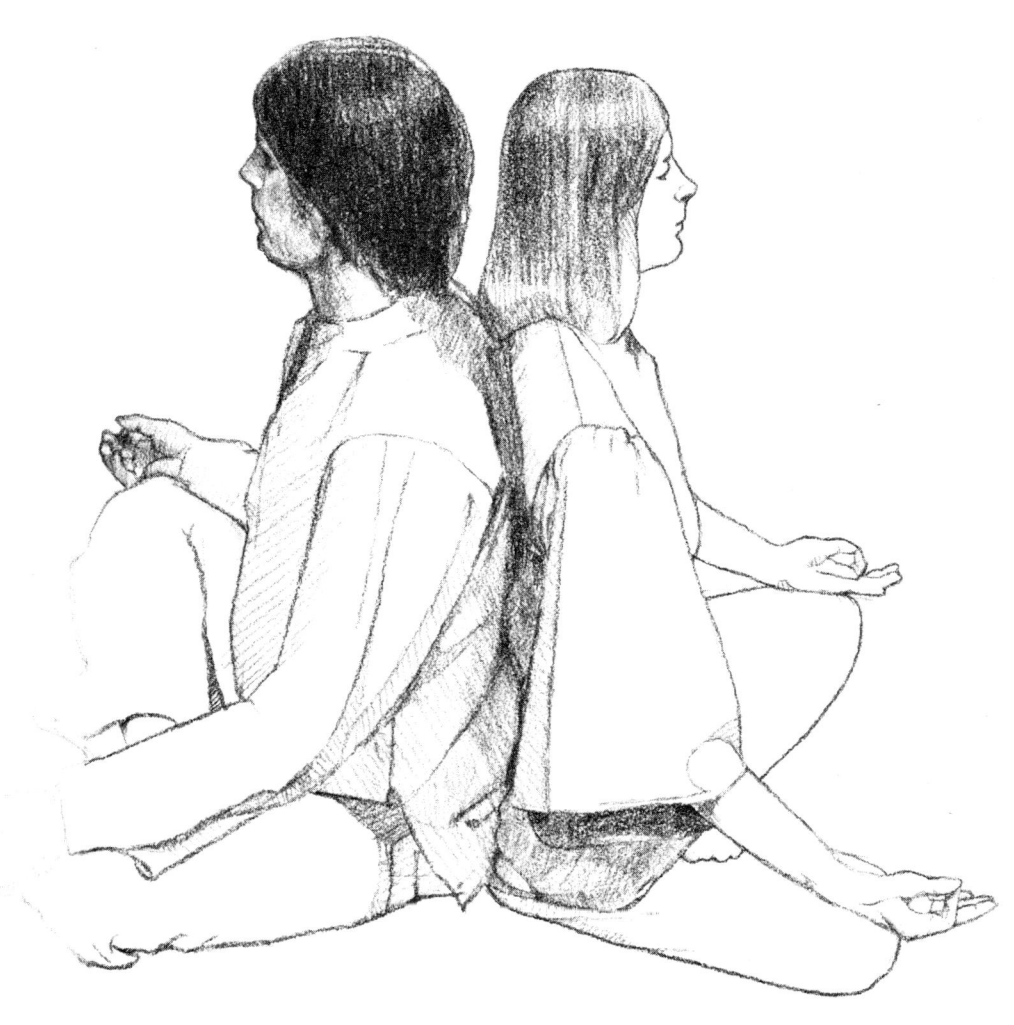

29. Meditate with Mantra Time: 5–15 minutes

Sit facing or back to back, and chant a mantra together.

One mantra often used for white tantric practices is the Sarab Shakti Mantri, an eight-part mantra listing the qualities of the Divine; it is thought to help break up negative samskaras (habit-patterns) and clear the magnetic field.

Gobinday	Sustainer (all peaceful)
Mukunday	Liberator
Udharay	Enlightener (who lifts us up)
Aparay	Infinite (who carries us across)
Haring	Creator/Destroyer (who is all and everything)
Karing	Doer (the ultimate doer of everything)
Nirnamay	Nameless (formless)
Akamay	Desireless

Variation: Repeat the mantra alternating syllables and coordinating the breath in reverse (each partner exhales upon speaking).

Group Practices

Tantric yoga techniques are suited more for couples than for groups, but, if properly used, they can be adapted for use by larger groups. Tantric yoga can raise group consciousness so that the group may become a better vehicle for spiritual growth. Small spiritual communities may wish to set aside several hours once or twice each week for practice; spiritual groups that are not communities might set aside one night each week to get together.

Groups may practice both in lines (with individuals facing each other) and in circles.

In linear formations, a group composed of couples would do best to line up by pairs. In groups without couples, individuals may rotate until each person has paired off with every other person (or with as many others as possible). If possible, one person who is not paired off should direct the group.

Circular exercises involve standing, sitting, or lying in a circle with the hands joined. In the same way that techniques for couples blend the auras of the partners, circular techniques create a group aura.

The closer to a perfect circle the group's pattern is, the easier the energy will flow. Also, if individuals are alternated male-female, as nearly as possible, the energy will flow more easily. When people stand or sit in a circle with the hands joined, the energy of the group will begin to flow around the circle. (There must be no break in the hands, or the flow will stop.) Hands are held so that the palms face the palms of the people on either side. A continuous stream of energy should be visualized flowing around the entire circle. Concentrate on drawing energy in from the left palm (feel the heat), up the left arm, to the heart. Then move the energy down the right arm and out the right palm. The group energy can be circled more and more powerfully so that it builds up like a dynamo.

The power generated by group techniques can be contained within the group for the purpose of consciousness raising, or it may be projected out as healing energy.

30. Stand in a Circle
Time: 5–10 minutes

Stand in a circle with the hands joined and the eyes closed. Tune into the circular energy flow.

31. Heads Together in a Circle*
Time: Unlimited

Lie down on the back, with the heads touching and the legs pointing outward, and join hands. Concentrate on circulating the energy. Chanting will enhance this process.

* Note: This pattern works best for five or six people. Larger groups can be separated into several circles, or else one large circle can be created, with only the shoulders touching (heads will not touch: there will be an empty space in the center of the circle).

32. Sit in a Circle
Time: 5–15 minutes

Sit in a circle, with hands joined and eyes closed. Sing, chant, or work with ideations such as projecting energy from the heart into the center of the group aura.

Variation: Meditate in a Circle
   Release hands and meditate.

Variation 2: Gaze across a Circle
   Open the eyes and gaze at the person directly opposite you.

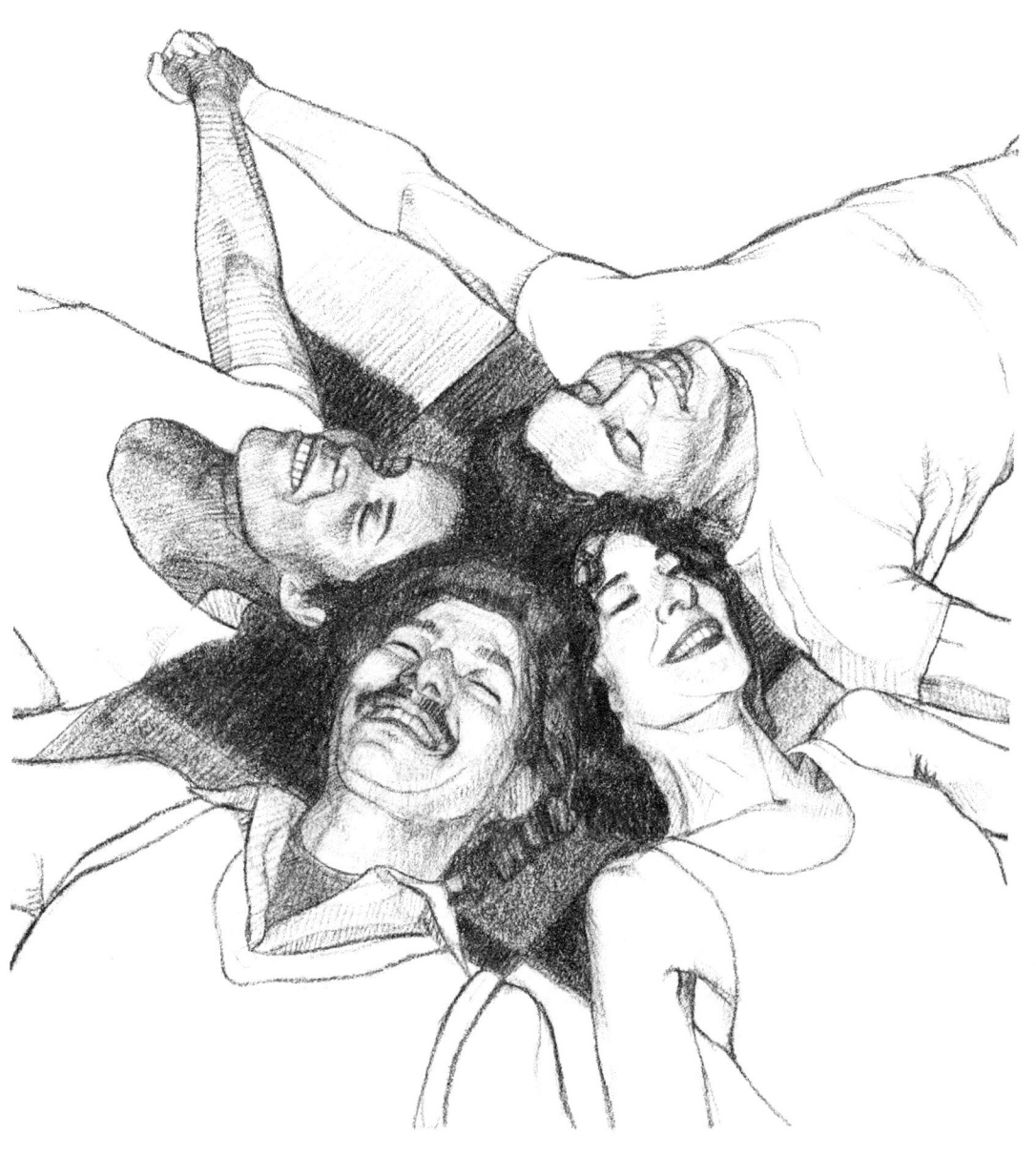

Glossary

Agni pranayam—See *pranayama*.
Apana—See *prana*.
Asana—"Posture," "positions," or "sitting": the asanas are the body postures of yoga.
Atman—Can be translated as "Soul" or "True Self," but literally means "the principle of breathing" or "the principle behind actions."
Aura—Refers to that part of the subtle body which extends beyond the surface of the skin.
Bhastrika—See *Pranayama*.
Chakra—"Wheel": The chakras are the innumerable energy centers of the subtle body. The seven major chakras are located along the spine, from the base of the spine to the crown of the head.
Hatha yoga—"Sun-moon" union (referring to the joining of the positive and negative energies): That branch of yoga which concentrates on physical culture.
Kapalabhati—See *pranayama*.
Kriya—"Action": yogic purification processes, and/or yoga techniques.
Kundalini—"The coiled one": the fundamental life force of the individual, which is normally latent (inactive). The traditional image of the kundalini energy is a coiled serpent which "sleeps" in the bottom chakra. Kundalini yoga aims to "awaken" the kundalini and raise it up the central energy channel so that it may activate the higher chakras.
Manas—"Mind," or literally "of man": the subtle substance of the thinking mind.
Mudra—"Seal" or "lock": refers to certain types of body postures which "seal" the pranas in the body and to certain hand positions which help to "fix" or "lock" the mind steady during meditation.

Nadi—"River": The energy channels in the subtle energy body which conduct the prana throughout the body.

Prabhupati—See *sadhana*.

Prana—"Primary energy": all of the energy in the universe, or, more specifically, the energy in the air and the energy that runs through the subtle body. Also, positively charged energy, as opposed to negatively charged prana, or *apana*.

Pranayama—"Energy control": yoga breathing exercises that aim to control the energy flows in the subtle body. This book describes natural breathing, yogic long, deep breathing, and two types of *Agni pranayama* ("fire breathing"):

1. Kapalabhati—"the shining of the skull": a breathing technique usually done at a rate of one breath per second; exhalation is forced and inhalation is passive.

2. Bhastrika—"bellows": a breathing technique usually done at a rate of three breaths per second; both inhalation and exhalation are forced.

Radhana—See *sadhana*.

Sadhana—"Accomplishing" or "fulfilling": the activities that constitute one's spiritual practices; in particular, the set of practices that constitute one's daily meditation/yoga set. The word *sadhana* is also used in the more narrow sense of the first stage of "discipline." The second and third stages of sadhana are *radhana* ("attitude" or "habit") and *prabhupati* ("mastery").

Samskara—"Impression": patterns of thought or feeling, mannerisms, et cetera—the subconscious impressions from the past that manifest as predispositions or habits.

Subtle Body—The energy body or the energy field; the nonphysical human body which contains the nadis and the chakras.

Vajrasan—"Thunderbolt posture": the simple yoga posture of sitting on the heels.